T0292221

Fascial and Membrane Technique

For Elsevier:

Senior Commissioning Editor: Sarena Wolfaard
Development Editor: Kim Benson
Production Manager: Jess Thompson
Project Manager: Andrew Davidson, Prepress Projects
Design direction: Judith Wright
Cover design: Stewart Larking

Fascial and Membrane Technique

A manual for comprehensive treatment of the connective tissue system

Peter Schwind

Director, Münchner Gruppe, Munich, Germany
Advanced instructor, Rolf Institute of Structural Integration, USA
Translation by Y²K Translations

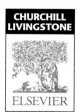

CHURCHILL
LIVINGSTONE

ELSEVIER

EDINBURGH LONDON NEW YORK OXFORD PHILADELPHIA ST LOUIS SYDNEY TORONTO 2006

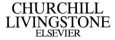

CHURCHILL
LIVINGSTONE
ELSEVIER

© 2003 Urban & Fischer Verlag München · Jena
English translation © 2006 Elsevier Limited. All rights reserved.

No part of this publication may be reproduced, stored in a retrieval system, or transmitted in any form or by any means, electronic, mechanical, photocopying, recording or otherwise, without the prior permission of the Publishers. Permissions may be sought directly from Elsevier's Health Sciences Rights Department, 1600 John F. Kennedy Boulevard, Suite 1800, Philadelphia, PA 19103–2899, USA: phone: (+1) 215 239 3804; fax: (+1) 215 239 3805; or, e-mail: healthpermissions@elsevier.com. You may also complete your request on-line via the Elsevier homepage (http://www.elsevier.com), by selecting "Support and contact" and then "Copyright and Permission".

ISBN-13: 978-0-443-10219-6
ISBN-10: 0-443-10219-8

British Library Cataloguing in Publication Data
A catalogue record for this book is available from the British Library.

Library of Congress Cataloging in Publication Data
A catalog record for this book is available from the Library of Congress.

Note
Neither the Publisher nor the Author assume any responsibility for any loss or injury and/or damage to persons or property arising out of or related to any use of the material contained in this book. It is the responsibility of the treating practitioner, relying on independent expertise and knowledge of the patient, to determine the best treatment and method of application for the patient.

The Publisher

your source for books,
journals and multimedia
in the health sciences

www.elsevierhealth.com

Working together to grow
libraries in developing countries

www.elsevier.com | www.bookaid.org | www.sabre.org

ELSEVIER   BOOK AID
                International   Sabre Foundation

The
Publisher's
policy is to use
**paper manufactured
from sustainable forests**

Printed in China

Cover image © Susanne Kracke, München
Photographs Susanne Kracke, München; photographs 7.9–7.14
Dr Sebastian Schmidinger, Seefeld Hechendorf
Illustrations Gerda Raichle, Ulm

Contents

Foreword to the German edition

I have known Peter Schwind for a long time; we first met seventeen years ago. Since that first meeting, we have been constantly engaged in a prolific exchange of ideas. Again and again we have asked ourselves how we can structure our work as effectively as possible so as to achieve the best outcomes for our patients. We have been guided by the fundamental concept that every aspect of the organism is important and we must not neglect a single one of its elements. This overarching philosophy of osteopathy served as a connection between us from that first moment and, over time, we discovered that we have much in common in our view of the human body.

Starting from my own work, particularly with regard to the diagnostic approaches of general listening, local listening, and manual thermodiagnosis, which I consider so very important, Peter Schwind has developed his personal research and way of treating patients. He has found new emphases within these areas and, in so doing, has elaborated on my own ideas.

It is his habit to work hard; he has a broad range of interests and approaches all things with curiosity. He is able to refine individual techniques with personal involvement and perseverance. In his practice, he works with a high level of commitment and he is an inspiring teacher. Everyone who meets him encounters the earnestness and passion which he applies to his profession.

For all these reasons it was a pleasure for me to write this short foreword to one of his books.

In practice, our primary duty is to be there for our patients and to help them. However, it is also important to teach and to write books such as this one. In so doing, we are able to make the little that we know accessible to a larger audience; we foster the sort of critical dialogue that is essential for the continued development of our field.

Peter Schwind is one of the therapists providing the drive behind this development. I am certain that he will continue to make a contribution to the progress of manual therapy in the future as well.

I thank him for having written this book.

Jean-Pierre Barral, DO
Grenoble, February 2006

Foreword

It is a pleasure to introduce the unique synthesis of Dr. Peter Schwind to the English-speaking reader. The book in your hand represents a significant contribution to the growing realm of what we could term "spatial medicine"—the study of what can be accomplished through the modification of shape.

Within the discipline of spatial medicine, some have concentrated on modifying articular mobility via thrust or other techniques, while others have focused on training or resetting muscle tone through manipulation, positional release, or exercise. More recently, the plasticity of the fascial interface between the muscles and the skeleton has received more therapeutic attention—namely the treatment of myofasciae, tendons, ligaments, and the many fascial membranes.

All these specific fascial structures, however, begin as a unitary three-dimensional "spider web" in the early embryo. Although the complex origami of development creates the illusion of separate structures, all these strings, sacs, and sheets are still part of a unitary matrix which continues to communicate bodywide throughout life. Thus they need to be considered as a whole, not piecemeal.

By combining the work of Jean-Pierre Barral in the visceral membranes of the ventral cavity, the insights of osteopathy concerning the spine and the dorsal cavity membranes around the nervous system, and the work of Dr. Ida Rolf on the parietal planes of myofascia, Dr. Schwind presents a complete picture that first unites and then transcends the source material to create an approach that is uniquely original.

The material within can perhaps be best understood through knowing that Dr. Schwind was, prior to his long career in manipulative therapy, an excellent musician. His sensitivity to the instrument and to the music itself has informed his many forays into the specifics of manual therapy. Over the years of our occasional acquaintance, I have observed Dr. Schwind explore the details—osteopathic techniques, dental work, visceral manipulation—with characteristic zeal and precision, but always with an eye to the "feel" of the whole piece, the entire gestalt of the client. With this book, he rises from musician to conductor, and I am as eager as anyone to have this seminal book available to me and to my students in the English language.

In manipulative therapy, nothing is subtracted but strain, and nothing is added but information. Thus, effective treatment rests on two elements: the ability to "listen" to the tension patterns, and the quality of the information the therapist can impart. While the quality of "listening" is difficult to impart in a book, Dr. Schwind does an excellent job of inviting the practitioner to participate "within" our clients, rather than "on" them, or doing therapy "to" them.

Pay attention, please, to the early chapters. The proper application of the manifold techniques offered in the body of the book rests on his approach to the "music" of the membranes. Absorbed from this point of view, this book will contribute significantly to the ability of any therapist both to understand the inner harmonies of the human body and to improve his or her skill at plucking the right strings in the right order.

Thomas Myers
Walpole, Maine, USA
October 2005

Acknowledgements

I would like to thank Jean-Pierre Barral DO for the many years we have worked together in our practical research on the nature of fascia and membranes. As a teacher, as a colleague and as a friend he has created an atmosphere of creative investigation for me and a group of colleagues in Munich, by sharing his vast clinical experience, showing an open mind, and stimulating the creativity of his colleagues.

I would also like to express my gratitude to several individuals, who have inspired me in my work on the concept of fascial and membrane technique. They all have contributed, sometimes by practical exploration of techniques, often by conceptual dialogue, and occasionally by productive disagreement.

In the United States my many thanks go to Jim Asher, Emett Hutchins, Peter Levine PhD, Jon Lodge, Jeff Maitland PhD, Peter Melchior (deceased), Stacey Mills (deceased), Tom Myers, Michael Salveson, Louis Schultz PhD, Bill Smythe, Jan Sultan, and Tom Wing.

In Brazil to Monica Caspari and Pedro Prado.

In Europe to Elmar Abram, Jean Arlot DO, Harvey Burns, Alain Croibier DO, Dr. Bruno d'Udine, Dr. Hans Flury, Dr. Laura Gentilini DO, Dr. Michel Ginoulhac, Hubert Godard, Anne Koller-Wilmking, Didier Prat DO, Robert Schleip, Dr. Sebastian Schmidinger, Christoph Sommer, and Pierpaola Volpones.

Chapter 1

Introduction

It has been a century since A.T. Still, one of the pioneers of the manual treatment of the human body, first noted the significance of the fascial system. Initially, his view of the comprehensive significance of this type of tissue was not seriously considered; however, an increasing number of approaches were being developed in which the individual aspects of this tissue were revealed in greater detail. During the 1930s, the science of anatomy focused on the fascial layers of the neck region for the purpose of discovering the transmission paths for certain pathogens. Later, as research began on the function of connective tissue within the immune system, the role of connective tissue overall attracted much more interest. However, the layers of connective tissue and their special formations, the fasciae, were given far less attention than the classical areas of the musculoskeletal system, organ systems, and nerve sys-tems. The role played by connective tissue for and between these three individual systems was little known.

In spite of the excellent topographical work that has been accomplished up to now, even today many anatomy textbooks contain only a marginal discussion of connective tissue for the purpose of clearly representing the details of the body. In these textbooks, most of the fasciae and numerous membranes remain unnoted, considered unimportant filler material. Although this limited description has some use in certain branches of medicine, it also contributes to a narrowing of perspective, in which our models of the human body are taken as objective reality and therefore the viability of other models with other classification schemes and points of view is ignored.

In the meantime, the science of anatomy has shown us that connective tissue for each of the systems mentioned above has clearly describable functions. It is known that it is just as present in the epimysial and divisional layers of the musculoskeletal system as in the fascial envelope layers of the organs and in the perineurial sheets of the nervous system. Histology is able to show the presence of connective tissue ranging from large areas of subdermal tissue to the periosteum and the smallest units of the cell. Thus, we now have enough information to understand the functions of each of the various layers of connective tissue within one bodily system. We can see how the fascial system surrounds individual muscles, divides them, and connects them to the periosteum by way of the tendons. We can see how membranes extend from the interior of the cranium by way of the dura mater and perineuria into the finest arborizations of the nervi nervosum. And it is therefore possible for us to construct an overall blueprint of the body as an interlaced system of connective tissue chambers.

This sort of analysis and classification therefore provides insight into the functions that the connective tissue performs for the anatomically defined subsystems. We also know which general functions the connective tissue performs for metabolism and the immune system. However, it is still unclear how connections between the individual subsystems arise and how the connective tissue as an organ of form provides the building blocks for these connections in the overall mosaic of the body (Varela and Frenk 1987: 73–89).

The techniques described in this book apply to the outer and subdivisional layers, whether within the musculoskeletal system, the organ system, or the nervous system, or, if we choose the traditional osteopathic classifications, within the parietal, visceral, or craniosacral region. The goal of treatment is to produce physiologically expedient mobility between the individual components of a region.

If we achieve greater mobility in one region, effects will also be felt in the other regions. In the practice of fascial and membrane treatment, the three-dimensional interconnection of fasciae and membranes means that the effects of a manual intervention simply cannot be limited to one individual subsystem of the body. Mobilization techniques, as soon as they are applied to the connective tissue system, are always a process that changes the shape of the whole organism as well. However, most examination procedures, in particular the mobility tests taught in manual schools, relate only to the subsystems; therefore there is an information gap about the way a single subsystem constitutes shape regarding the interconnection of the systems to one another in practice as well.

If treatment is restricted to the subsystem alone, i.e. if the detailed technique is used without a more "global" intermixing, then the therapist must rely on the greatest precision. The effectiveness of this sort of procedure lives and dies by the diagnostic precision of the assessment of the subsystems and the "minimalistic selection" of treatment steps.

I am of the opinion that this very efficient concept of mobilization of precisely describable units shows its limitations as soon as we turn our attention to the bridging, interconnecting function of fasciae and membranes mentioned above. Fasciae and membranes are the medium of interaction between the individual systems of the organism; not only do they function within the individual systems, but they also serve as "mediators" between the various systems of the organism.

The techniques described here address this mediating function. Although these techniques do apply to the various individual layers of those aggregates that we called parietal, craniosacral, and visceral, they should also be applied, as far as possible, to the broader, more global interrelationships of form.

First of all, fascial and membrane treatment should be understood only as a technique. I have tried to depict the practical applications in such a way that they may be used in various manual

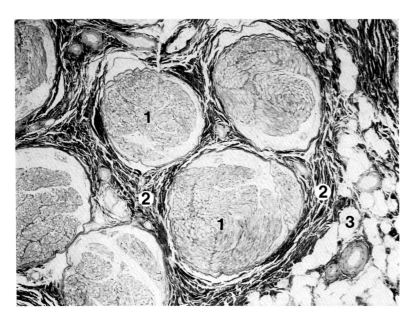

Figure 1.1 Cross-section of the n. ischiadicus (enlarged 300 times, photograph by Klaus Siebert, Anatomical Institute of the University of Hamburg). 1, nerve fibers; 2, connective tissue; 3, fatty tissue.

disciplines. However, behind the technique as well as its numerous variations in application, there is one unified concept. I have made an effort in some cases to describe the technique with such meticulous precision that this concept shines through. It is a concept that, on the one hand, is based on the basic osteopathic theme of mobilization that is as precise and as gentle as possible and, on the other hand, ties in with the form-stabilizing approach of Ida Rolf's *Structural Integration*.

This conceptual emphasis may best be clarified as follows:

How, practically, should we proceed so that we can treat details in a precise manner and, at the same, have an effect on the larger form with its global interrelationships? One answer to this question may be found in the treatment of mobility restrictions in the ribcage: we treat the small components that may be found in the interior of the cavity in such a way that, at the same time, we are influencing the organization of the exterior form. Thus, for example, it is possible to influence an adhesion of the pleura with subtle pressure while, at the same time, the intercostal membranes and the deep fasciae are incorporated into the treatment as well.

A second answer may be found in the treatment of the segmental organization of the leg. We treat the details of the muscular fasciae, the intermuscular septa, and the interosseus membranes in such a way that a positive effect occurs on the fine tunic structures of the nerves and thus an improved neural function is supported.

The nerve is the river; the fasciae, membranes, and perineurial envelopes form the riverbed. In order to ensure a better equilibrium of flow in the river, we treat the riverbed.

Chapter 2

Fundamentals

Terminology

The term *fascia* is used in anatomical literature for the envelopes and separating layers of musculature that are composed of connective tissue. In a narrower sense, fasciae consist primarily of collagen connective tissue, the fibers of which intersect in a latticed pattern (at 45 degrees). The tough collagen fibers are also combined with true elastic fibers to varying degrees (Waldeyer and Mayet 1993: 29; Benninghof 1994: 169).

Fascial tissue has the ability to return to its original form after deformation, and this is largely due to the combination of elastic and collagen fibers within it. The collagen fibers have a tendency to return to their original configuration that is reinforced by their cooperation with the elastic fibers. The proportion of collagen and elastic fibers within any area of fascia depends upon the functional demands placed upon the tissue in that area. If there are strong tensile stresses on the tissue, then the collagen portion will predominate and there will be fewer elastic fibers. If the shape of a segment of the body changes repetitively, then the equilibrium shifts toward the elastic fibers, which in this case will partially replace the collagen fibers. The fascial system is thus able to adapt to changing functional requirements of the body over an entire lifetime. This adaptive capacity is not reduced until old age, when the proportion of elastic fibers within the interstitial matrix decreases, and the tough collagen fibers predominate more and more.

In a functional approach to the musculoskeletal system, it is not possible to discuss the fasciae separately from the muscle fibers to which they belong. There is no muscle tone without a corresponding tensing of the fasciae and no tensing of the fasciae without muscle tone. Anatomy refers to this inseparable interconnectedness as "myofascial unity."

Yet there are also layers of fasciae with an astonishing independent dynamic that can hardly be caused by muscular activity. These layers connect to the periosteum of the bone by ligaments with no intervening musculature. One example is the lower section of the lumbar fascia. It forms a thickly interwoven unit with the sacroiliac ligaments on the posterior side of the sacrum and, via the sacroiliac ligaments, connects with the periosteum of the sacrum.

The investing, differentiating, and supporting functions of normal muscular fascia will vary as we move toward the origins of muscles. The tensile forces increase as we approach the origins, and this gives rise to an aponeurotic compacting of the tissue. However, even these compact fascial structures, like the "normal fascia" of muscles, have a sliding layer, the epimysium, beneath them.

The term *fascia* is often used in anatomy also for layers such as the endothoracic fascia—a very fine layer consisting largely of *loose connective tissue*. The endothoracic fascia displays the typical fibrous structure of fascia only in its uppermost region, at the level of the pleural cupula. The endothoracic fascia has a completely different function to that of the muscular fascia in that it enables the parietal pleura to slide in relation to the inner thoracic wall.

The term *membrane* is used in anatomical literature for various types of connective tissue. Examples include the dense, two-dimensional fibrous membranes that connect individual bones, e.g. the interosseus membranes of the extremities, as well as annular elements such as the atlanto-occipital membrane.

In osteopathic literature, the term *fascia* is used almost synonymously with *connective tissue* (see Friedlin 2003).

Although such usage cannot be entirely justified from a histological point of view, its almost universal acceptance has a certain validity. The various forms of connective tissue—the tunic layers of organs, the ligamentous and membranous connections between bones, and their associated sliding layers—all perform the same function despite their structural differences: functions such as the regulation of the maintenance of shape and the possibility of motion between single components. Most types of connective tissue perform these functions in a similar manner and therefore are comparable to the fasciae in the narrower sense of the word. Moreover, there is a continuity, a global interconnectedness, between the various forms of connective tissue. Individual bands, such as the retinaculae of the ankle joint, are simply local concentrations of fibers of fascia, in this case as part of the crural fascia of the lower leg. In a certain sense, therefore, bands may also be understood as a specialized form of the fascial and membrane system.

Material properties of connective tissue

All connective tissues typically provide the organism with both a flexibility and a connective stability because they are composed of certain intercellular materials as well as cells. The totality of these intercellular materials is referred to in anatomy as the *extracellular matrix*. This matrix is composed of collagen and elastic fibers as well as ground substance. The material properties of the various forms of connective tissue depend greatly on the proportion of the fiber and ground substance within this matrix. Collagen and elastic fibers have entirely different material properties.

Collagen fibers can usually be stretched only up to 5 percent of their length.

Elastic fibers do not display any ordered structure, and are visible in electron microscopes as an amorphous mass. They consist of elastin, in which microfibrils are embedded. Their elasticity arises from the structure of the elastin itself. It is composed of interconnected protoelastin molecules so arranged that they can be lengthened and yet return to their original length. Elastic fibers can be reversibly stretched up to 150 percent of their length. Within this range of extension, they return to their initial length; however, if they are extended beyond this, i.e. beyond 150 percent of their initial length, then a long-term deformation of the elastic fibers occurs. This means that connective tissue which contains a high amount of elastin is particularly susceptible to processes of deformation. To a certain extent this explains the plasticity of connective tissues. Hence an irreversible overextension of certain fibers will have a long-distance effect on other areas of the organism, since changes in tension are transmitted throughout the interconnected system of the entire fascial network.

The material properties of elastin are responsible for the transmission of tensional forces, along with collagen fibers, which have a more limited flexibility. If tension is applied to collagen fibers, they are pulled from their crimped rest position into a linear extension. If this force is reduced, then elastic forces come into effect; the initial tension of the collagen combines with the elasticity of the elastin to pull the fibers back into their crimped rest position. In loose connective tissue the amorphous intercellular gel, *ground substance*, plays a role in this process by allowing the sliding of adjacent surfaces. Ground substance has a high water-binding capacity and, besides its so-called fixed cells, also harbors free cells that are able to wander throughout the tissue. This is particularly important in the sliding movements of the organs during the motion of breath.

Muscular fasciae contain very little of the loose types of connective tissue, but much more of the formed components of the intercellular matrix: the slightly flexible collagen fibers and the more flexible elastic fibers. The fibers arrange themselves according to how tensile forces act on the stiff connective tissue. If the tensile forces come from several different directions, then a woven arrangement of fibers is typical, as is found in the fasciae of muscle tissue for instance. If instead only linear forces are applied to the tissue, then the fibers will align themselves in a parallel fashion, as can be seen, through the microscope, in the slightly crimped alignment of the fibers that form tendons. When longer-term heavy stresses are applied to the tissue, then the stiff collagen increasingly supplants the elastin. The denser tissue layers then become more able to resist strain, but in the process become less adaptive as some of the elastic quality of the elastin is lost.

Small elastic bridges may also be found in tissues that are chiefly inelastic. This can be found, for example, in the interface between tendons and bones. The tendon is not affixed directly to the bone, but rather is glued to the periosteum by a fine layer of connective tissue.

Consequences for treatment

The wide range of material properties found in the diverse forms of connective tissue has definite implications for treatment. Because all connective tissues develop in an environment of variable stresses, it may be that the same fascia with the same topographical location has completely different properties in two individuals. Different patterns of stress will create quite distinct and individual distributions of the collagen, elastin, and fluid components. For this reason, it is not possible to establish any absolute rules for the treatment of individual fascial and membrane layers, although certainly there is a basic technical orientation that is valid. So, for example, layers containing elastin require a subtle treatment, whereas layers containing a large amount of collagen can tolerate quite intensive pressure. As a rule, however, even in the case of the stiffest fasciae with a very high proportion of collagen, there will be a sliding layer separating it from the muscle fibers, which contain a considerably larger amount of fluid. We must also take this sliding layer into account when treating relatively inflexible layers of fasciae. In practice, a proven procedure is to apply pressure obliquely to the surface of the skin in order to press gently through the tender layers and affect the deeper sliding layer.

The significance of the tensegrity model

The term *tensegrity* refers to a construction principle that may be traced back to R. Buckminster Fuller. He developed it following the work of Kenneth Snelson.

The term is a portmanteau of the two words "tension" and "integrity" (Myers 2001: 41–50).

The idea underlying this structural principle is that certain kinds of stable, adaptable forms can be achieved chiefly through the transmission of elastic tension. This structural principle was first used in architecture, with elastic elements defining the links between the solid components. However in

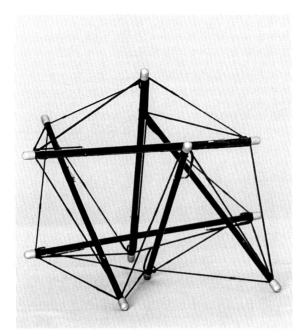

Figure 2.1 Tensegrity model consisting of solid and elastic elements.

tensegrity structures there is no direct contact between the solid components—unlike, for example, the solid components that form a stone wall (Horwitz 1981: 5–8).

In tensegrity structures, the interconnection of solid and elastic elements creates a three-dimensional spatial puzzle. If external forces are applied to this puzzle, then the entire system reacts with an adaptive redistribution of tension. These external forces are thus distributed throughout the system, modifying the preexisting patterns of tension within the system. As this redistribution of forces occurs, a greater stability emerges through the interactions of the stable and elastic elements under stress.

The tensegrity model was already applied to the human organism two decades ago on the basis of the drafts presented by architecture within the teaching of Ida Rolf's *Structural Integration*. This model has recently developed a large resonance within osteopathy as well (Meert 2003).

In recent years, the tensegrity model has begun to be identified as a universal schema of form in biological structures. Donald E. Ingber has convincingly demonstrated that the tensegrity model

is also well suited to describing the blueprint of a cell (Ingber 1998).

If the tensegrity model is used to describe the structure of the human body, i.e. at the level of its macrostructure, close parallels with the architectural construction principle can be found. The human organism appears as a dynamic combination of solid parts, the bones, and the elastic parts, the myofascial layers and membranes that wrap the bones. In many ways, this simple schema describes the movement of the human body far more reliably than traditional arthrology. It clarifies the fact that the transmission of force in the human organism does not occur from solid body to solid body, but rather is conveyed by way of elastic bridges. However, in comparison with architectural tensegrity constructions, the tensegrity construction of the human body is far more complex. The basic plan, the combination of solid and elastic elements, is similar to the basic plan of an architectural construction. This basic plan could be called the "rough structure" or the "myofascial skeleton" and can be described in a relatively simple manner. However, within this basic plan there is an additional "internal structure" built into the human body. Upon closer inspection of the fascial and membrane system, we find a variety of elastic and movable microelements within the ground substance that act as buffers between the relatively solid collagen fibers. In contrast to the simple tensegrity model, the human body has sliding surfaces separated by liquids. Additionally the body contains a series of hydrostatic chambers that are partially or entirely sealed off, as we find in the large body cavities.

The tensegrity of the human organism is therefore a complex system consisting of tensile effects, the sliding behaviour of individual elements, the state of their surfaces, and the liquid films that separate them. This is both a three-dimensional network and a system of sliding surfaces whose elements have varying degrees of elasticity.

Consequences for treatment

Such a differentiated structure has significant consequences for treatment practice. The tensegrity model explains why one section of the body may be treated with fascial and membrane techniques without its being directly touched. Because of the continuous nature of the fibrous network of connective tissue, corrections may be made in one place that affect different areas entirely.

This also provides a new perspective for looking at the function of joints. If we observe that the transmission of pressure through joints is always cushioned by elastic or liquid elements, then obviously we need only direct some of our attention to the bones in diagnosis and treatment.

With the aid of the tensegrity model, it is easier to understand that components located far from the individual joint may have an influence on it. Because all fibers are interconnected, the force acting on a joint may be transmitted to parts of the body that have no muscular connection to the joint at all.

Consequences for the technical and practical side become apparent as well: if it is actually true that all components are connected to one another and that even strongly connected components are embedded within an overall elastic context, then it must be possible to treat these consolidated connections using a low or relatively low amount of force. For example, if one of the metatarsal bones is massively limited in its movement relative to the adjoining bones, the correction of this problem would normally require a very quick impulse with a low degree of movement and a high-velocity, low-amplitude impulse. If instead we use the properties of the tissue, the larger context of fasciae and bands, we need only a relatively low expenditure of force. Such a procedure combines the treatment of significant details with the effect on a larger interconnection of form and may be expected to produce a more lasting result.

Plasticity: the malleability of connective tissue

Fasciae and membranes respond to the forces acting through them. Therefore, they are not simply the passive filler tissue that is sometimes described in anatomy. The dynamic growth properties of the fascial tissue of the mature human being hark back to the early stages of embryonic development. As cartilage forms within the embryo, forces act on the collagen fibers adjoining the cartilage in a specific direction. This causes a parallel alignment and a compacting of the fibers. This process allows the attachment of tendons to bones that will later develop in the embryo. In the later stages of development, a similar process occurs in the formation of the myofasciae. During the growth and development of the muscle fibers, the muscular fascia (or myofascia) receives mechanical stresses that align its fibers in certain directions. The typical lattice fibers of the muscular fascia usually tend to align in a transverse direction relative to the line of pull of the muscle. This occurs because forces are exerted in a variety of spatial directions. This weave-like arrangement allows cooperation with the sliding layer, or epimysium, and the fascia and muscle fibers as the muscle changes its form. Here, the relatively large proportion of fibrous connective tissue in the muscle fascia acts as a spatial boundary allowing it to be stretched only up to a very limited extent.

If a change in volume acts on a fascial layer over a large surface, as we may observe in the thorax during breathing, more elastic fiber and fluid elements of the ground substance are integrated into the fascia. This process is evident if we look at the morphological structure of the endothoracic fascia.

Immediately after birth, as the child is taking its first breaths, a stretching impulse is exerted on a large area, indeed on all the intermediate layers of the thorax wall. In this process, the endothoracic fascia functions as an elastic sliding element between the thoracic wall and the parietal pleura, which closely adjoins the visceral pleura and thence the lung. Two-dimensional expansive forces are exerted during breathing and this induces the endothoracic fascia to develop into a relatively thin, elastic layer. Peculiarly, it has a different material consistency in only one small section. This section is located in the uppermost region of the pleural cupula where the endothoracic fascia covers over the bulges of the cupula. In this area, the endothoracic fascia has a higher proportion of fibrous layers and therefore has properties reminiscent of a muscular fascia. These features do not arise by chance. In the uppermost section of the endothoracic fascia, in the region referred to in the literature as *Gibson's fascia*, tensile forces are constantly at work. There is a direct connection between Gibson's fascia and the cervical spine by way of a band-like divergence of tissue from the scalene fascia. As the scalene muscles contract and raise the upper ribs, an essential part of the breathing process, rhythmic tensile forces act upon the upper part of the endothoracic fascia. The fascia reacts to this unified, directionally dependent tensile effect by aligning its fibers and partially replacing the elastic portion of the fibers with inelastic collagen fibers.

This example shows how the functional exertion of forces can have a lasting structural effect on the morphology of an individual fascial layer and can induce different kinds of tissue structure within the same fascia depending on its function. The fibrous, less elastic layer in the uppermost part of the Gibson's fascia is consistent with the tensile mechanics that act in the superior direction at every intake of breath and with the small changes in volume that occur there. The thin, elastic layers of the fascia in the middle and lower thoracic region, however, are richer in fluids, and are more consistent with the manifestly large changes in respiratory volume that occur there; this thoracic expansion has a two-dimensional effect on the fascia in addition to the tensile forces that have a relatively small effect there.

These adaptations occur over a long period of time. The exterior form of the body is in a process of constant change through the processes of new tissue formation, fiber realignment, and changes in the hydration of the connective tissues.

Consequences for treatment

In treating the fasciae and membranes, we try to influence this process of adaptation and encourage it in a particular direction. We influence the tissue so that its inherent self-regulatory tendency is reinforced in a direction that is more appropriate to its function. In a way, therapy ought to accelerate the ongoing, long-term processes of functional adaptation. Experience suggests that our therapeutic interventions can lead to immediate changes in the pattern of tissue tensions. Tension patterns are simply the spatial interlacing of various fascial tensions; they persist despite superimposed muscle activity and postural changes. Thus, besides long-term processes of adaptation, there appears to be a direct change of tension in the fascial network that is more or less irreversible.

The example of whiplash

The rapid reshaping of a stable tension pattern can be seen in a fairly extreme form in the case of whiplash injury (see Chapter 8). In this injury the fibrous portions of both the fasciae and the membranes of various components of the organism are rapidly overextended within a fraction of a second. The collagen fibers, which have limited flexibility, absorb a large portion of the energy. If bone fractures occur, however, much of the energy is absorbed in the process of the break. Curiously, in the case of these severe bone injuries fewer overextensions of the myofascial layers tend to occur, whereas the same process without fractures leads to more permanent and severe effects on fasciae and membranes. In such cases, the fibers containing elastin are overextended by a multiple of their initial length in some places and are only partially able to return to the original tension pattern. Subsequently, severe long-term effects may be expressed symptomatically, for example, with headaches, neck discomfort, and vertigo. Interestingly, permanent changes to the form of the organism can result from traumas with a relatively small forces acting on the body. It is not so much the magnitude of the forces but their direction that is responsible for the changes in the tissue. In other words, even a relatively small force can cause significant deformities if it acts from a particular direction on fascia that contains elastin, particularly if that fascia normally stabilizes various elements of the body.

This process is easier to understand if we apply the tensegrity model. The structure of the body is remarkably stable when we consider the interconnected nature of its solid and elastic elements. If even one structurally vital element has its elastic consistency irreversibly changed, a very sustained process of adaptation spreads throughout all the parts and therefore alters all spatial relationships. We often find that the organism then strives to find a new equilibrium.

It should be stated again: the overextension of fibrous connective tissue may be found not only in high-speed traumas but also in cases with a relatively low-speed impact. One possible explanation for this may be found in the different material properties of the fasciae and membranes. For each fascial and membrane layer, there is a threshold value of the return forces acting through the elastin.

This threshold value is high in layers that contain a large proportion of collagen and is correspondingly low in layers with a large proportion of elastin. If the mechanical force is greater than that threshold value and impacts the corresponding layer, then a drastic deformation will occur and the tissue will be unable to return to its neutral initial position.

I think that the form-altering effects that manual therapies can have on connective tissues parallels to a certain degree the effect of forces involved in whiplash. In this sense, the therapeutic effect can be seen as a "whiplash" divided into small and carefully applied steps, each with a positive presymptom. It acts locally through lengthening the tissue. However, this lengthening will modify tension patterns only if the extension threshold value of the elastic layers is exceeded.

In practice, this means that, while applying a technique, the therapist must constantly monitor the changes in tension at the contact points in order to modulate the intensity of the contact according to the organism's response.

This entire process is a complex one, and research so far has yielded only some of its features. All manual therapies are applied to the skin, but we don't really know how this contact affects the skin and its connection to the subdermal connective tissue and the tiny, honeycomb structures of the subcutaneous fatty layer and their bridges to the deep fascia. We can be certain, however, that the organism reacts to the contact. While the patient is lying, apparently passively, on the treatment couch, the patient's nervous system is highly active.

Recently, research has attempted to view this activity of the nervous system during therapeutic treatment in a new light. Robert Schleip has summarized the research approaches and thus arrives at a new interpretation of the plasticity of the fasciae (Schleip 2003: 20–8).

Schleip correctly refers to the presence of mechanoreceptors in the fascial system and to the possible significance of the interstitial receptors and Ruffini's endings to myofascial treatment. He emphasizes the connection between fasciae and the autonomic nervous system in general. In this sense, fasciae are "outposts" of the autonomic nervous system.

In this scientific research, there are numerous references to this kind of a link between the autonomic nervous system and the fascial and membrane system. In therapeutic practice, the long-lasting effect of treatment of fasciae on the autonomic nervous system is known.

If the initial findings of the research into the inherent contractility of fasciae are borne out, this would lead to an entirely new view of the term *plasticity*. In this manner, we could arrive at a broader view of the biomechanical significance of fascia and membrane techniques. A.T. Stills' speculative statement describing the fasciae as "branch offices of the brain" would thus be confirmed.[1]

---

[1] Cited in Schleip; see there as well the compilation of research literature.

Chapter 3

Principles of treatment in practice

In the curricula of most forms of manual therapy training, the discussion of therapeutic setting (or therapeutic environment) is usually regarded as of secondary importance, and this is in marked contrast to training in psychotherapy. This disregard of therapeutic setting does not reflect the challenges that confront manual therapists in their day-to-day practice. From a traditional viewpoint, the therapist is the expert, the active "subject," who treats the (possibly quite uninformed) patient as if he or she were a passive "object." There is certainly a kernel of truth in this viewpoint because the hands of the therapist actually do stimulate the organism of the patient in such a way that preexisting impulses are guided in other directions and, in a certain way, new objective realities are created. These new objective realities may include, for example, verifiable changes in the movement path of a joint, improved gliding behavior of layers of tissue adjacent to one another, and improved fluid exchange between body cavities. Yet this viewpoint does not take into account the fact that manual treatment involves a multilayered communication process that is similar in many respects to psychotherapy. In modern practice, this important fact is increasingly ignored as the use of physical devices has begun to shape the normal course of therapy. We do not wish to discuss here how effective or ineffective these devices are or how specifically or unspecifically they influence the body. This type of critical question may be asked only in the context of empirical studies. However, it is a legitimate and important question for anyone engaged in day-to-day practice to explore the manner in which this "hands-free" treatment differs from treatment in which the hands of the therapist are used. The use of medical devices that administer mechanical, electrical, or electromagnetic impulses may, for example, locally or globally alter the muscle tone or provide stimuli to the nervous system in a clearly defined manner. However, such devices are unable, or able only to a very limited extent, to register the response of the organism at the same time as they administer the impulses, to process the response as feedback, and to use this feedback to durably modify the impulses being administered. The stimuli of these devices are therefore fundamentally different from the stimuli originating from the human hand. The difference lies in the fact that the human hand is able to vary its stimuli using feedback from the brain in an almost infinite variety of ways, and therefore is able to register the responses of the organism being treated while it administers the impulses. To put it differently, the hand may be used simultaneously to transmit and receive information; the hand provides a stimulus and, at the same time, registers the effect of this stimulus on the organism of the patient. In order to allow this process to take place, a series of preconditions for the therapeutic setting must be taken into account.

In order to make use of both aspects of touch, transmission and receipt, i.e. administration of the impulse and observation of the response, the therapist must depend on being able to switch freely between an active and a passive use of the hands. We will see that, for certain techniques, it is possible and even necessary for part of the hand to be actively engaged while another part of the same hand behaves passively. This sort of differentiated use of therapeutic contact can succeed only if the therapist is able to guarantee a "neutral" setting.

This "neutral" setting, the therapeutic setting, is characterized by some basic rules of communication.

Internal equilibrium of the therapist as a basis for observation

In order to be able to observe the patient with as few outside influences as possible, it is necessary

for the therapist to be neither in an overactive state nor in a too-passive one. In this state, both poles of the therapist's autonomous nervous system, the ergotropic and trophotropic sides, are equally activated. As soon as the therapist emphasizes one side, this emphasis will be transferred to the patient through the quality of the contact. In this manner, the internal state of the therapist is intertwined with the overall state of the patient, making an objective diagnosis no longer possible.

Presence of the therapist

In order for the spectrum of observation to be as broad as possible, the therapist must be completely present mentally. During the application of diagnostic or therapeutic techniques good coordination is essential.

Efficient therapeutic contact is characterized by the fact that it is sensitive enough to detect the most minuscule differences in surface characteristics while at the same time registering the condition of components that are distant from the immediate point of contact and that may be detected only through the interconnection of the three-dimensional fascial network.[1] Differentiated attentiveness lends a sensual quality to the contact. At the same time, however, it is important to maintain an "objective" or neutral quality to the contact. Only in this manner is a specific and precise impulse effect possible.

To a certain extent, therapeutic contact has paradoxical qualities. On the one hand, it adapts very gently to the form of the body and thus automatically attains an expressive character, for example, in the sense of support, friendliness, or a positive prevailing mood. On the other hand, therapeutic contact should also be distanced without producing callousness or giving the impression of emotional detachment.

This paradox can also be seen in the basic communicative role of the therapist. The therapist should simultaneously express closeness through the physical contact with the patient but yet remain at a friendly distance as a person. This can be best described by the following image: the hands of the therapist are very close to the organism while the

---

[1] This ability is widely referred to as "end-feel."

therapist's self is distant from the personality of the patient. Only in this manner is it possible to produce a therapeutic setting that, to some extent, corresponds to Sigmund Freud's working principles. In the context of this setting, the therapist will hardly be influenced by the patient's own moods and feelings. Only within such a setting is the therapist able to efficiently control the course and efficacy of the therapy.

Therapeutically efficient contact

It is extraordinarily difficult to document scientifically what occurs during the manual treatment of the human organism. Part of the difficulty lies in the fact that human contact always manifests itself in the organism on completely different levels at the same time. And whenever we observe one level in isolation, there is the danger that we will take into account only a partial aspect of the investigation or even "measure" a pseudoresult. In addition, contact always has an individual quality. The quality of contact may be similar in different people but ultimately is always individual, like the handwriting of two different people. However, it is still possible to formulate a kind of basic technical orientation that may be valid for the most varied types of contact.

I have already referred to the fact that every human contact unites in itself two aspects. One aspect may be characterized as passive and non-directive—this means to observe, to diagnose—and the second may be characterized as active, directive, and providing a stimulus—this means to actually treat. Many forms of treatment attempt to separate these two aspects from one another to the greatest extent possible. They use the non-directive, passive side of contact for diagnosis and the active, directive side for precisely defined manipulations. I think that this kind of separation is not entirely realistic and, moreover, carries with it increased risks in treatment. Every form of human contact in the therapeutic realm should unite directive and non-directive qualities. In other words, one of the aspects can move more into the forefront while the other aspect retreats into the background and vice versa. This means that the passive/non-directive aspect is present throughout the entire treatment

and not only during the diagnostic process. In this manner, it is possible for the directive impulses originating from the therapist's hand to be modified in such a way that they utilize forces already at work in the organism of the patient and therefore are more effective and gentler at the same time.

The use of the hand-contact technique

The first and generally applicable distinction for the practical use of the hand is the distinction between weight and active pressure. As soon as the therapist's hand is placed on the surface of the patient's body, the weight of the therapist's hand, forearm or upper arm, and shoulder is transferred onto the body of the patient. The therapist can intensify this weight, for example, by leaning forward over the axis of the hip and adding the weight of the torso. In this case, the coordination of the therapist plays a large role in the quality of the contact. Finally, the contact becomes more effective as soon as the therapist uses active, directive pressure in addition to the applied, passive weight.

In the treatment of fascial and membrane layers, it is essential that we train our own perception so that we can clearly differentiate between the various forms of contact. When the patient is lying on his or her back and the therapist's hand is placed on the surface of the patient's body, the weight of the therapist's hand and forearm is transferred onto the body of the patient no matter how carefully the therapist is making the contact. The therapist's hand being placed supportively under the patient's back however is a completely different process. In this case, the weight of the therapist's hand and forearm is transferred onto the treatment couch and the patient's weight is transferred to the therapist's hand and forearm. Both forms of contact have a different quality, reach different levels, and are perceived by the patient as two fundamentally different ways of being touched.

The most efficient treatment techniques for the fascial and membrane system use both forms of touch at once. The therapist can thus use one hand dorsally to support the patient lying on his or her back, i.e. to accept the weight, while using the other hand ventrally to work with weight and/or active pressure. The therapist is therefore literally taking the organism in his or her hands. This allows the therapist to give consideration to the entire three-dimensional network from the outset instead of receiving just a selective, linear, or superficial impression.

Another important distinction is the difference between stationary, local contact and sliding contact. In sliding contact, the speed must be adapted to the tension of the tissues; the denser the fibers, the slower the contact must be.

The next step toward technical differentiation of contact is the differentiation between the use of the palm and the individual fingers or the thumb. A large number of possible combinations are available in practice. Despite a widespread misunderstanding, the palm is much more sensitive than the fingertips in differentiating fine distinctions. For this

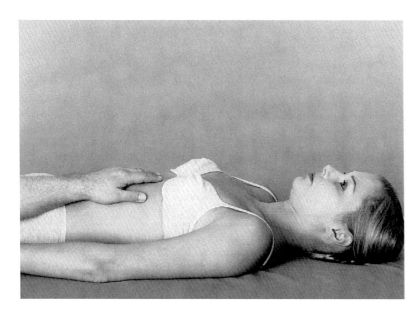

Figure 3.1 Contact with the deep fascia using the weight of the forearm and hand.

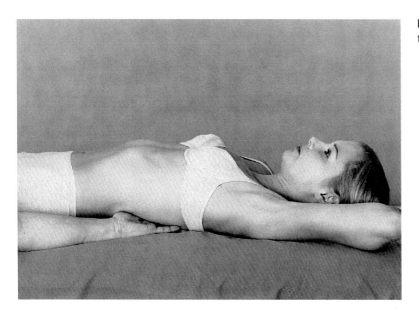

Figure 3.2 Supportive contact with the deep fascia.

reason, the combined use of the palm and the fingers is particularly efficient when the palm is used in a supportive and observational capacity while the fingers provide an active stretching impulse.

Another differentiation of contact is made possible by the fact that each of the fingers can be used to apply a different amount of force and can apply stretching impulses in different directions independently from one another.

The most important technical condition for being able to treat the fascial and membrane system efficiently in its spatial structure is the independence of one hand from the other, the independence of the palm from the fingers and thumb, and finally

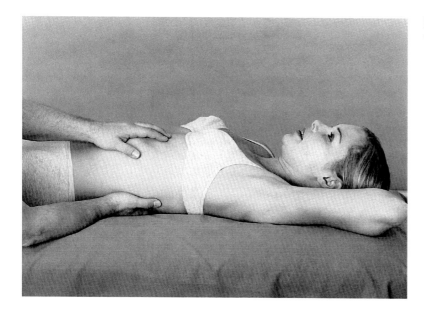

Figure 3.3   Combined contact: use of weight (ventral) and support (dorsal).

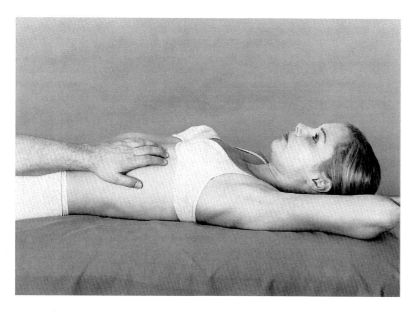

Figure 3.4   Combined contact of the fingers and palm.

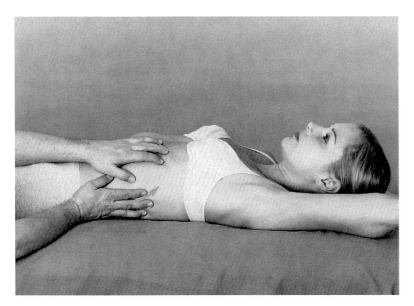

Figure 3.5   Simultaneous stretching impulses in different directions.

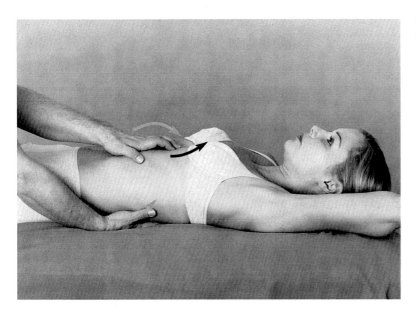

Figure 3.6   Treatment of the deep fascia to the side of the sternum.

the independence of the individual fingers and thumb from one another.

Direct application of the fingertips in the region of the deep fascia

The therapist initially places only sufficient weight on the fingertips to allow him or her to reach through the skin and the subcutaneous fatty layer to the deep fascia. The base of the fingers is then lowered somewhat so that the fingertips contact the surface of the body diagonally. When the therapist relaxes the musculature of the pectoral girdle and upper arm, more weight is applied to the fingertips. At the moment when this increase in weight acts on the deep fascia, the therapist applies an active stretching impulse by extending the fingertips a little more.

This technique lends itself to the treatment of the deep fascia of the torso.

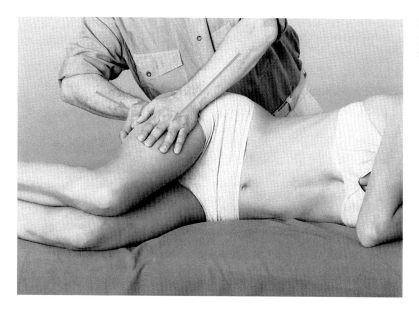

Figure 3.7   Direct application of the palm in the region of the lateral section of the fascia lata.

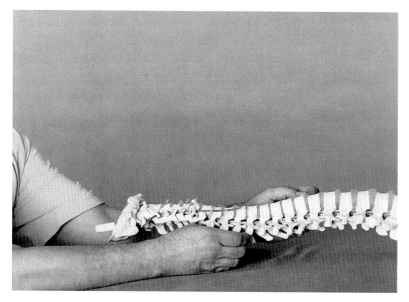

Figure 3.8   Indirect application of hands resting on their sides in the region of the posterior intercostal membranes.

Direct application of the palm

The palm is primarily suitable for direct stretching application to layers with a large surface area. In this technique as well, it is important to note that contact is made with the deep fascia by way of the skin and subcutaneous fat. The palm adapts to the form of the structures present below the superficial fascial layer. This technique can be performed using the weight of the hand and forearm as well as with additional active pressure. As soon as the palm has reached the relevant layer of the deep fascia, a slow, stretching impulse is applied in that the palm slides parallel to the bone located beneath this layer. In this process, it is important that active pressure be applied either parallel or perpendicular to the bone so as to not overextend or crush the tissue.

In order to perform this process successfully, it is usually necessary to support the patient dorsally with the other hand.

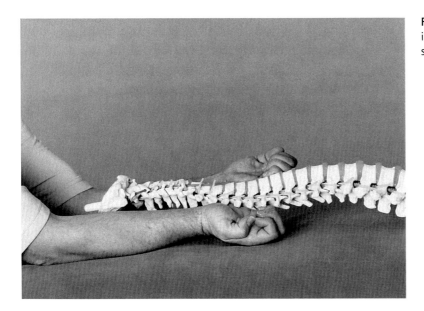

Figure 3.9 Indirect treatment of the intercostal membranes and the subcostal myofascial units.

Indirect application of the medial edges of both index fingers

The therapist places both hands on the treatment table in such a way that the outer edge of the hand and the little finger transfer weight onto the table. With the lateral edges of both index fingers, the therapist accepts the weight of the body part to be treated. The contact is gradually adapted to the surface form and finally to the interior form. Then, while "listening," the therapist follows the dominant direction of pull.

This contact technique is appropriate for the treatment of the dorsal intercostal membranes.

Indirect application of the backs of bent fingers of both hands

It is possible for the therapist to vary the preceding technique by placing the back of both hands and the elbows flat on the treatment table and bending the fingers in such a way that the patient comes to rest precisely on the foremost finger joints. In this case as well, the contact of the individual finger joints is initially adapted to the surface and then to the inner form that can be felt below the surface until clear directions of pull emerge. The therapist follows these directions of pull by "listening" while supporting the larger form with the balls of the hands.

This technique is appropriate for the treatment of the dorsal intercostal membrane and the myofascial layers of the subcostal musculature.

Direct application of the second phalanges over small areas

The flat contact of the second phalanges of the index and middle fingers is suitable for the treatment of tough layers of tissue. The therapist applies pressure in order to directly influence the muscular fascia by stretching.

Application of the first phalanges for direct stretching over large surfaces

In order to use this technique, the therapist forms a fist only far enough that no blunt pressure contact results, but rather an elastic effect is maintained, or the fist is held open. The therapist takes care that his or her wrist does not bend as soon as weight or pressure is applied. The transfer of force should occur more or less in a straight line from the forearm to the first finger joints. Only when the therapist has gently used the contact to access the deep fascia through the surface layers does the therapist begin to slide perpendicular to the fiber direction with a strong contact.

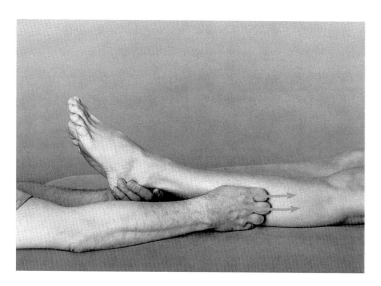

Figure 3.10   Direct treatment of the fascia of the long peroneal muscle.

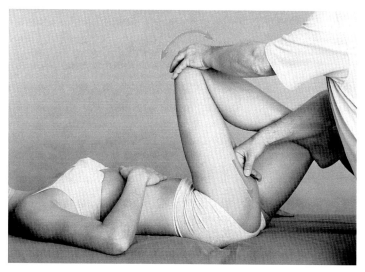

Figure 3.11   Contact with the first phalanges for the direct stretching over a large surface of the posterior section of the fascia lata.

In using the technique with a closed fist, care must be taken that the fist is only gently clenched. For this, an imaginary aid can be helpful; the therapist imagines that a small object is enclosed inside his or her fist. The intent of this technique is therefore not to press into the tissue with a stiff fist, but rather to keep the hand gently closed so that a surface contact is produced with the first phalanges. This surface contact is most effective when the therapist uses primarily upper body weight, keeps the shoulders relaxed, and applies only a small amount of additional pressure. Care should be taken as soon as the therapist has arrived at the fascia through the surface layer and intensifies the contact. The speed of the sliding must be modified in relation to the reaction to the tension of the tissue. If individual sections of tissue have a firmer structure, the speed of sliding should be reduced. However, at these points, the therapist continues to slide with very intensive pressure, only more slowly. At points that are elastic, the therapist can increase the sliding speed somewhat, but still remains in strong contact. This technique is primarily suitable for fascial layers that cover a large area, especially in the lower extremities and the back.

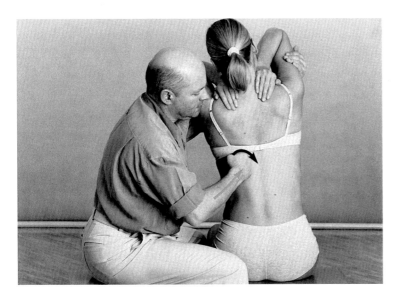

Figure 3.12 Contact over a large surface in the region of the fascia of the latissimus dorsi.

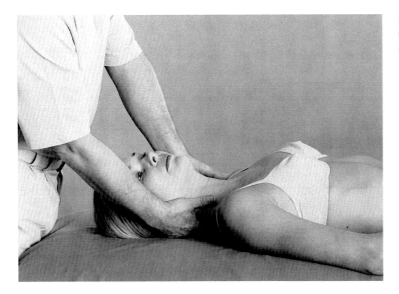

Figure 3.13 Two-dimensional application of both palms in the region of the fascia coli superfiscialis.

Two-dimensional application of both palms

The two-dimensional application of the entire surface of the hand and fingers is primarily suitable for the treatment of the superficial layers of the neck and the transitional layers between the upper thoracic cavity and the lower cervical region. The contact should be made in such a way that the longitudinal vessels are not compressed. In order to do so, the contact should be kept two-dimensional and should not translate into exterior sliding on the surface of the skin. The sliding that is used is actually only a stretch of a few millimeters in which both of the therapist's hands should be moved slightly toward one another without forcing the neck as a whole into a stronger flexion or extension (see Upledger and Vredevoogd 1983: 54–5).

Selective contact in the treatment of small membrane units

The application of contact to small tissue units requires a precise approach, almost at a single point. This procedure is primarily suitable for the

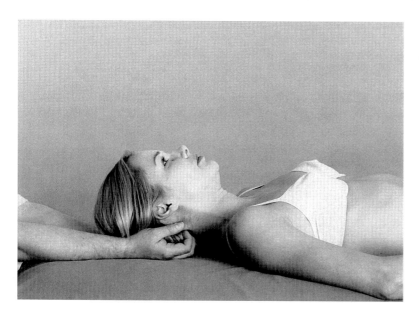

Figure 3.14 Selective contact for affecting the posterior section of the atlanto-occipital membrane.

treatment of transitional areas in the organism, which naturally have a narrow structure, e.g. for the treatment of the transition between the posterior section of the neck and the base of the skull. The deciding factor is that the fingertips remain in contact with the lowermost edge of the occiput of the cranium, the palms very gently support the back of the head at the same time, and the foremost phalanges actually point vertically to the ceiling. They should not exert any active pressure but rather simply support the weight of the head and thus act on the suboccipital layers. If applied correctly, this type of contact acts initially on the muscular connections between the axis, atlas, and occiput and, if the therapist waits patiently, also on the membrane layers located in the region of the foramen magnum.[2]

Global contact with membrane layers in the interior of the cranium and/or vertebral canal

In traditional craniosacral osteopathy, which works with Sutherland's flexion–extension model, very subtle pressure of only a few grams is used. Techniques may be used to supplement this procedure that produce more intensive contact with the membrane system. In the treatment of the entire path of the dura between the cranium and sacral bone, the therapist maintains slightly elastic and, at the same time, strong contact with the base of the skull and the frontal bone. The tensile behavior of the dura mater of the spinal cord and the structures connected to it may be diagnosed and influenced using this treatment.[3]

Although the mode of functioning of this technique emphasizes the interior membrane system in the area of the head and spine, it has a drastic effect on the surface structures as well. It is only too easy for us to forget that, even when we are treating deep membrane structures, our hands first come into contact with the skin and the layers close to the skin of the organism. The technique described above affects not only the falx cerebri and the tentorium cerebelli but also the galea aponeurotica, which is rich in sensory and motor nerves.

Combined contact with the body stocking and structure of the thoracic cavity

Given the three-dimensional interconnection of the fascial and membrane system, the manual influence

---

[2] Upledger has made reference to the fact that this technique also affects the foramen jugulare and thus the cranial nerves that pass through this foramen. see Upledger and Vredevoogd (1983: 58).

[3] The tests that must first be performed before this treatment are described in detail in Barral and Croibier (1999: 184–90).

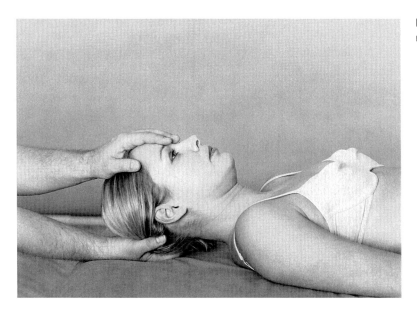

Figure 3.15 Global contact with the membranes of the craniosacral system.

on one individual fascial layer always has side-effects in producing broader spatial consequences as well. Techniques that are not only selective, linear, or two-dimensional, but rather are applied in a three-dimensional, spatial manner from the outset, have a particularly long-lasting effect. One example is the simultaneous treatment of the body stocking and deep membrane layers in the region of the thoracic cavity. The therapist produces a contact with one palm on the front side of the thoracic cavity by literally modeling the cur-vature of this section of the body. At the same time, the therapist's fingertips are anchored in the body stocking. Because the therapist's palm is now slightly compressing the ribs, the therapist can then influence the sliding behavior of the membrane layers located between and beneath the ribs. While doing so, the therapist maintains strong contact with the deep fascia and applies an active stretching impulse in places where compacted fibers are noticeable. While doing so, the therapist's other hand is supporting the same rib region from the posterior side. Here as well, the form of the therapist's hand is adapted to the individual form and grips into the thoracolumbar fascia. If this technique is applied correctly, it is possible to treat simultaneously the body stocking and deep membrane structures that occur on the anterior and posterior surfaces of the thoracic cavity. In this manner, the tension patterns underlying the exterior and interior form are treated at the same time.

Indirect application of both hands for the treatment of the interosseous membrane of the lower leg

In order to reach the interosseous membrane in the lower leg, the therapist places both palms dorsally below the upper and lower thirds of the calf. The lower leg should be resting in both of the therapist's palms in such a way that the therapist is able to support its entire weight while the fingers still have room to move. The therapist now also dorsally contacts the medial edge of the fibula with the fingertips of one hand and the medial edge of the tibia with the fingertips of the other hand. While both palms continue to support the weight of the lower leg, the fingertips attempt to reach as close as possible to the periosteum of both longitudinal bones. The indirect efficacy is now possible because the therapist is following the tension of the membrane by "listening" through the fingertip contact and is keeping both hands sufficiently relaxed that the contact points move toward one another in the direction of tension of the membranes until relaxation occurs.

Indirect application of the fingertips to the periosteum of the bone

After a fracture has healed, a compression of the bone tissue and the surrounding periosteum occurs

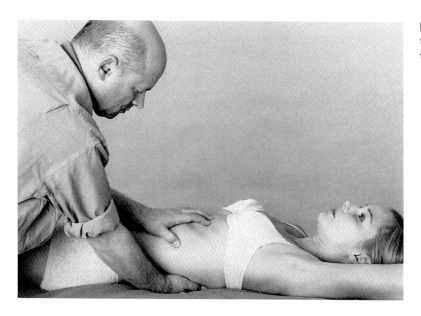

Figure 3.16   Combined contact with the body stocking and structure of the thoracic cavity.

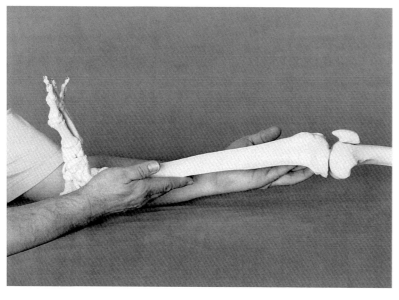

Figure 3.17   Indirect application of both hands and the fingertips to the interosseous membrane of the lower leg.

at the break point. The treatment of this type of tissue compression requires a special application of the fingertips and the thumb. This technique, which can be used for all bones of the extremities as well as on the sternum and collarbone, is indirect. The therapist surrounds the bone on both sides of the break point with the tips of the fingers and thumbs of both hands. In so doing, the therapist is definitely in contact with the periosteum but avoids holding the bone stiffly in place. By "listening" and following, the therapist exaggerates only very slightly the

inherent tendency of bones to bend in on themselves after a fracture. At the same time, the therapist intensifies the contact between the two contact points as if to displace the periosteum slightly from its connection to the bone.

Direct application of the ulna to the large ligaments of the pelvis

The application of the ulna makes it possible to produce an extremely strong contact with tough

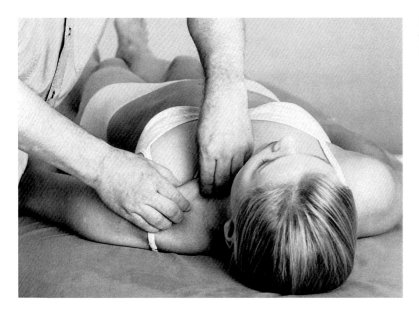

Figure 3.18 Indirect application of the fingertips of both hands to a healed collarbone fracture.

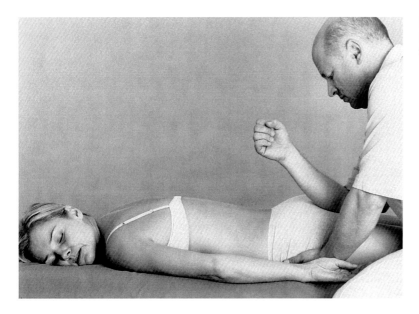

Figure 3.19 Direct application of the ulna to the region of the sacrotuberous ligament.

structures. It is primarily suitable for the treatment of larger myofascial units and for the treatment of the larger ligaments of the lower pelvic region. It is important to ensure that the ulna does not have strong contact with the patient's tissue until it has arrived at the layer in question. For example, in order to affect the sacrotuberous ligament, it must first make its way through the muscle layers located on top of this ligament. The best method for doing so is for the therapist to gradually apply more upper body weight to the ulna by way of the pectoral girdle and upper arm without additionally tensing the pectoral girdle or the upper arm. With some coordinated deftness, the ulna may be applied very intensively in this manner in that the therapist increasingly relaxes the musculature of the pectoral girdle and upper arm and almost exclusively uses body weight.

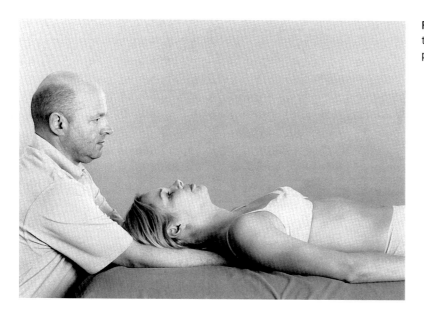

Figure 3.20   "Natural table" for the treatment of tension patterns in a psychoemotional context.

Support of the interior form in the region of the thoracic cavity: the "natural table"

The following type of contact can be varied in a number of ways. However, one consideration has fundamental significance: very deep components of the myofascial system and the membranes may be contacted only if patients are allowed to maintain a certain basic equilibrium in their exterior musculature that is typical or habitual for them. This basic equilibrium arises when their preferred postures have become obvious in their bodily form or structure. The therapist's task is to position his or her hands such that the patient can lie on them and maintain their preferred position of the back and thoracic cavity. In a certain way, the therapist's supporting hands reinforce the typical pattern of tension with the autonomic musculature of the patient's back and thoracic cavity. Thus the therapist's hands, forearms, and possibly upper arms form a "table" beneath the patient that allows the patient to rest in the position that appears "natural" to his or her. The deciding factor is that as many contact points as possible be available to the therapist for the construction of the "natural table." For example, this occurs when the occiput of the patient is supported on the one side with the therapist's lower arm, thus leaving the hand free to reach downward in the transitional region between the thoracic and lumbar spine while, on the other side,

the therapist's palm is supporting the base of the skull and the therapist's fingers are attempting to gain contact with the atlanto-occipital connection.

This form of contact and its variations are primarily suitable for the treatment of tension patterns in a psychoemotional context.

A comparable technique can be applied in the region of the pelvis and lumbar spine. One of the therapist's hands is supporting the interior curvature of the sacral bone and the other hand is supporting the curve of the lumbar spine.

Basic rules of fascial and membrane technique

In the section about the material properties of connective tissue (Chapter 2), we saw that connective tissue has a distinctive capacity for functional adaptation. It reacts to long-term strain from compressive and tensile forces. In this process, collagen fibers are organized into a functionally suitable arrangement while the balance of fluid content between the various fascial components will vary. However, the organism does not have a control system that can regulate this process precisely. In the longer term the body reacts to repetitive, monotonous motion by overcompensating. The compression and realignment of fibers, which at the outset is expedient, then develops dysfunctional

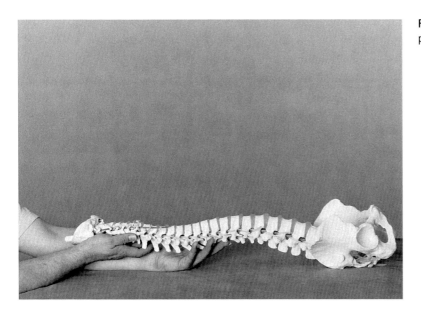

Figure 3.21 Clarification of the position of the hands on a skeleton.

properties; finally it will restrict mobility and encourage a defective exchange of fluids in the united cell structure. This process can occur in very different ways in individual cases. The aim of the techniques described in this book is to intervene in the overcompensation process and assist in regulating it.

In practice, the use of fascial and membrane technique requires an approach that is precisely differentiated on an individual basis. In spite of the vast range of individual specialized forms within the fascial and membrane system, it is still possible to formulate some basic rules that have proven themselves in practice:

- Overly tense myofascial layers of the musculoskeletal system require a direct lengthening; this lengthening is performed as parallel as possible to the muscle fiber and transverse to the primary fiber direction of the fascia.

- Slack myofascial layers of the musculoskeletal system are treated carefully and in a slowly sliding manner; the contact is broad and superficial, and linear contact and point loading are to be avoided.

- Band structures that create connections between bones respond well to so-called indirect techniques: the origin and connection

of the band are brought closer together until a motion impulse is sensed at the origination and insertion surface of the bone. In the case of large bands, e.g. in the region of the pelvis, an alternative strategy may be used: the therapist initiates a slow-acting impulse by contacting the middle section of the band while observing the reaction of the bone structures held by the band by "listening." It is important to avoid overstraining the band fibers.

- Interosseous membranes and deep septae respond best to subtle contact: therapy is performed indirectly here as well. It follows the dominant fiber paths, allows the bones to slide more strongly into their fixations, provides a gentle impulse to reinforce the fixation, and at the moment of strongest fixation then follows the releasing countermotion by "listening."

- Envelopes and ligamentous structures of organs must be treated carefully. These layers of tissue require a sensitive contact that takes into account the so-called turgor effect, the inner pressure dynamics of the organ, and its fluid dynamics. In the course of one treatment session, the applications must be limited to two or a maximum of three organ complexes in order to allow the organ system sufficient range for self-regulation.

- Elements of the craniosacral system may be treated with very different contact quality. In adult clients, it must be appreciated that each technique begins indirectly, that the structures affected are initially moved into a stronger fixation and only then—with constant "listening"—is a minimally corrective impulse applied with the aid of the momentum of the craniosacral system. This procedure—first indirect and then carefully direct—must also be observed in treating the exterior layers of the cranium such as the galea aponeurosis and the temporal fascia.

The overriding basic rule of fascial and membrane technique is to treat each fascia and each membrane in such a way that, by "listening," we take into consideration the three-dimensional interconnection of the overall system. In treating the more superficial layers, this means that we have to monitor the quality of our touch in a way with sufficient intensity that the deeper layers can follow the response of the superficial layers. For the treatment of deep elements within the extremities and body cavities, this means that we mobilize them only as far as their exterior perimeter containment gives room. Thus, while acting on smaller anatomical units as precisely as possible, we try to respect the overall form of the larger interconnection of tissues. This allows us to avoid provoking the body's resistance and prevents us from irritating the tissue to a large extent. And it is thus possible to improve the interior and exterior mobility while assisting the interior and exterior stability of form in the organism.

Chapter 4

Form-oriented treatment techniques

4.1 BREATHING

Breathing as the central force in the development of form

One of the central working hypotheses of fascial and membrane technique is that fasciae and membranes respond to steady or repeated strain by a gradual process of adaptation. This is described in the literature as changes to fiber orientation, fiber bundling, and the shift in the balance of connective tissue elements with a higher or lower fluid content. These steady strains arise from the compressive and tensile forces that act through constantly recurring patterns of movement. These movements become the driving force behind the development of the organism's form. They prompt a densification of individual groups of fibers that is at first functionally expedient but later leads to restrictions of movement and fibrotic tendencies of the tissue as soon as a certain limit has been exceeded.

For example, the breathing motion occurs over 20,000 times per day. This is the movement pattern that dominates all recurring forms of movement. Other forms of rhythmic movement parallel the constancy of breathing motion in certain respects:

- the cardiovascular motion originating from the heart muscle
- the rhythm of lymphatic motion
- the movement patterns that are summarized by the term "craniosacral pulse"
- organ motility, which was recently described by Jean-Pierre Barral (Barral and Mercier 1998, 2002; see also Chapter 6).

Like the breathing process, these forms of movement may be sensed in all areas of the body. However, they do not have the massive shearing force associated with breathing movement.

This driving force arises from the activity of the diaphragm, which is powered by the phrenic nerve, especially from the contraction of the diaphragm's lateral muscle fibers. At the same time, a countermovement occurs in the region of the upper ribs as they are raised by the action of the scalenes, the external intercostals, and the intercartilaginous muscles.

As the diaphragm contracts and the rib-raising muscles mentioned above become active, the

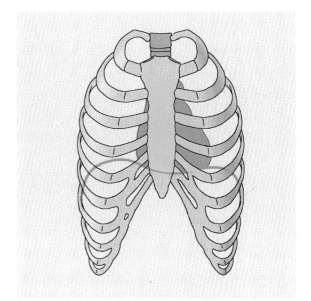

Figure 4.1   Exhalation position of the diaphragm and heart.

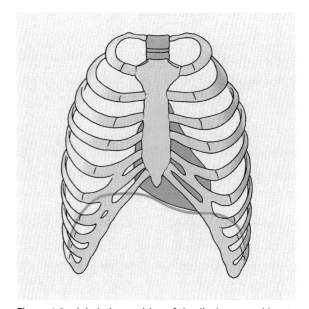

Figure 4.2   Inhalation position of the diaphragm and heart.

volume inside the chest cavity increases. In normal cases, i.e. when there are no drastic limitations to movement, this increase in volume spreads throughout the entire torso and causes a change to the exterior form of the torso that is synchronous with the breathing motion. This change in form may be seen in the back, where the curvatures in the spine tend to lengthen during inhalation. It is important to note here that, during inhalation, the muscle force acts in opposition to the elastic forces of the fasciae and membranes, whereas during normal exhalation muscle force has a very minor effect. The exhalation process occurs as so-called passive breathing, caused by the differences in pressure between the chest and abdominal cavities and the elastic resetting force of the fasciae and membranes of the ribcage in combination with the resilient effect of the rib construction. The only other active components are the internal intercostals and the transversus thoracis muscle. It is only in the case of extreme, forced exhalation that the body enlists the aid of the contracting force of the abdominal muscles.

Besides the obvious visible increase in volume in the chest cavity during inhalation, there are also changes in spatial relationships occurring internally: the diaphragm displaces the heart inferiorly (see Figs. 4.1 and 4.2) and exerts a downward pressure on the organs beneath it:

- intraperitoneal, in particular on the liver and stomach
- retroperitoneal, on the kidneys.

The liver and stomach are drawn on a spatial curve toward the navel during inhalation and return to their original position during exhalation. During inhalation, both kidneys move downward within the renal fascia, which is open in the medial direction, with its upper pole inclined in the anterior direction. The kidneys also return to their original position along a clearly defined spatial curve during exhalation. As Jean-Pierre Barral has persuasively described, the other organs of the abdominal and pelvic areas also participate in the breathing motion (Barral and Mercier 2002).

Barral chose the term *mobility* for the movement of the organs caused by breathing and developed a precise manual diagnostic repertoire for the evaluation of this movement and its limitations. In contrast, *motility* is a movement whose rhythm is independent of breathing (see also Chapter 6).

If we observe that there is an intraperitoneal excess of pressure compared with the chest cavity, it becomes clear that the entire ribcage is resting on the diaphragm as if on a trampoline that is curved upward toward the cranium. This trampoline, the

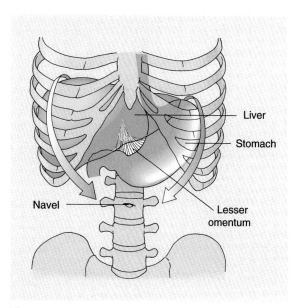

Figure 4.3 Mobility of the liver and stomach during inhalation.

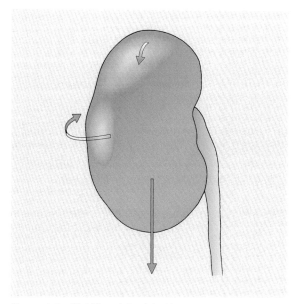

Figure 4.4 Mobility of the right kidney from the anterior direction during inhalation.

abdomen with the organ cavities located under it, forms the dynamic foundation of the ribcage.

The manner in which the abdominal cavity and chest cavity are connected to one another plays an important role in maintaining the entire torso erect. If limitations in movement occur for the

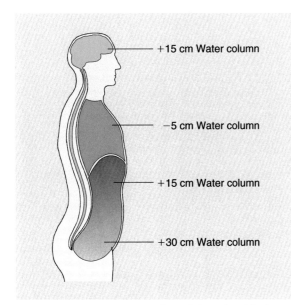

+15 cm Water column

−5 cm Water column

+15 cm Water column

+30 cm Water column

Figure 4.5 Average pressure values of visceral cavities in cm water column.

organs on one side of the diaphragm, the natural excess pressure in the abdominal cavity is unevenly transmitted to the chest cavity and an inevitable compensation occurs in the region of the thorax and pectoral girdle (see section 4.3).

These compensations may make themselves known in the most different sections of the fascial network within the chest cavity and have an effect on vertebral joints and costal vertebral joints.

> In the case of limitations of movement in the region of the thoracic spine, it is worthwhile first investigating and, if necessary, treating the transition between the abdominal cavity and chest cavity. In so doing, it is possible to avoid quite a few direct joint manipulations that usually bring only short-term relief.

When the chest cavity as a whole responds to movement restrictions in the diaphragm and the organs connected to the diaphragm, it has only a limited capacity to compensate and equalize because of its relatively stiff structure. The breathing motion requires a stable frame of movement in

the ribcage in order to guarantee the increase in lung volume. This frame of movement consists of components having various degrees of density and elasticity. At first glance, the ribs and spine, with their bony and cartilaginous elements, appear to form this stable element. However, a closer look shows us that the solidity of the bony arrangement can exist only in cooperation with the contents of the ribcage. If we were to remove these contents, only an extremely fragile bone structure would remain, which would give way under only a little pressure. The fact that the ribcage maintains the necessary level of stability arises from the manner in which the fasciae of the intercostal musculature and intercostal membranes respond to changes in interior volume and how they arrest forces acting from outside. Thus, it is not only the bones that provide a stable frame of movement for cardiac and pulmonary activity; rather, it is the cooperation of the various components that ensures the required combination of stability and mobility. In this area as well, fasciae and membranes are the form-stabilizing link between bones, cartilage, muscles, and organs. Here, too, they must guarantee adequate mobility of the individual components relative to one another in combination with sufficient stability of the overall form.

I have already mentioned that the changes in pressure and shear forces on layers of tissue that are directly related to the breathing process are particularly significant. The permanent presence of the breathing motion leads to local shortenings in the fascial system that are transferred to the three-dimensional structure of the fascial network, and thus initiates a compensation process that is quite complex spatially. This process may extend over long periods of time and often becomes evident from discomfort that occurs weeks or months later.

> A typical example of this is the oft-encountered progression of whiplash, which may cause only very little discomfort immediately after an accident, and does not become a problem until days or even weeks later.

This compensation process has its most lasting effects on layers located in or near the transitional zones of visceral cavities. The transitional areas between the abdomen and lower chest cavity and between the upper chest cavity and the neck area are particularly significant in this regard. If deviations from the norm occur in the fascial network in these regions or if changes arise in the direction of pull of individual membranes, a "displacement" of entire sections of the body relative to one another may occur.

If a limitation of movement occurs in the region of an organ located inferior to the diaphragm, the diaphragm is also affected by this limitation of movement. This process may be clearly observed in the case of reduced organ mobility of the stomach or the liver. The excursion of the half of the diaphragm on the side of the affected organ is reduced. The activity of the musculature between the ribs and the associated fascial layers and membranes responds to this change as well. As a result, a visible exterior alteration of form, as well as ultimately a tangible interior alteration of form, of the adjacent thoracic wall arises.

A similar process occurs in the region of the upper transition at the connection between the chest cavity and neck region as soon as form-stabilizing layers of connective tissue display an asymmetrical tensile behavior. Because there is a direct connection between the uppermost section of the endothoracic fascia and the transverse processes of the lower cervical vertebrae, increased tensile forces acting on the cervical spine from the upper chest cavity may limit movement of the affected joints. In advanced stages, this situation favors a tendency toward arthrotic changes.

> The endothoracic fascia is largely developed as a very thin layer. Only in the uppermost section, in the regions in which it envelops both pleural cupulas, is it distinctively dense and ropy. This natural thickening of tissue is a signal that the connecting ligament, which is joined with the scalene fascia and leads to the cervical spine, actually transmits tensile forces and functions as a suspension for the pleural cupulas.

Before we discuss the individual layers of connective tissue necessary for the breathing process, it will be helpful to analyze how the segments of the torso are connected to one another spatially.

Spatial relationships between the segments of the torso

The human torso is "divided" into chambers with various levels of hydrostatic pressure (see Fig. 4.5). These differences in pressure play a particularly important role with regard to erectness at the transition between the abdominal cavity and the thorax; higher pressure conditions in the abdominal cavity compared with the chest cavity press the organs in the upper abdominal region against the diaphragm and thus form a foundation for the ribcage, which is in constant motion. Without the excess pressure in the abdominal cavity, the liver and stomach would sink when a person is upright. This support function of the abdominal organ column would thus be lost and erect posture of the torso would no longer be possible. In contrast to the liver, the pyloric part of the stomach is very mobile and is constantly able to change its position in the abdominal area as soon as its weight changes because of the contents of the stomach or it is affected by displacement forces caused by turgor in another adjacent organ. Along with the pressure from the descending colon, the stomach can push the left half of the diaphragm so far upward that the diaphragm is almost horizontal and both of the diaphragm cupulas are arching almost symmetrically, which is a deviation from the norm. In addition, there is a very dynamic motion relationship between the diaphragm, spleen, stomach, colon, adrenal gland, and kidney on the left side of the body between the ninth and eleventh ribs. The spleen rests as if on a scale on the left phrenicocolic ligament, i.e. on the ligament that functions as the suspension for the left portion of the transverse mesocolon on the ribs. I have referred to the transition between the abdomen and thorax as an "upended trampoline." This "trampoline" is substantially more mobile on the left side of the body than on the right because the spleen provides a very dynamic "intermediate element." Even a small change in the position of the upper body causes the spatial displacement of this organ. In the same manner, the effects of pressure originating from a full stomach can change the spatial position of the spleen as well. So we can see that the spatial relationship between the abdominal and chest cavities is anything but static. The right diaphragm zone is the more stable element in this relationship, whereas the left half is more mobile and less stable, particularly because of the displaceable nature of the spleen and the "nested system" of the spleen, stomach, colon, adrenal glands, and kidneys. The diaphragm adapts to the pressure conditions of the upper abdominal cavity. This adaptation in turn causes a shear effect on the organs of the thorax. An example of this is the displacement of the stomach in the cranial direction, which causes pressure on the pericardium and is often misinterpreted by the patient as cardiac symptoms.

The outer parietal spatial structure of the pelvic, abdominal, and chest segments has in turn its own dynamic. There are certainly patterns of posture that arise again and again in various daily activities. These patterns are the dominant tensile pattern of the musculature and the fascial-membrane identity. This sort of tensile identity is determined substantially by the autonomic musculature, but also by the extent to which general muscle coordination allows the change from extension to flexion in the torso. People who always hold themselves in an over-erect position or who frequently sit or stand with a slouch are not only expressing the spatial relations of anatomical units. Rather, very specific preferred patterns of activity function as the "director" of the spatial units of the pelvis, abdomen, and chest. The manner in which the chest cavity rests on the abdominal cavity and on the pelvis is influenced by preferred patterns of perception as well as the tactile and visual orientation of the person in space. With regard to human locomotion, we know that there is a movement pattern that is present even before the beginning of the intended movement process. Hubert Godard referred to this process as anticipatory movement activity.[1]

[1] H. Godard, *Improvement of Sensory Dynamics [Verbesserung der sensorischen Dynamik]* in: P. Schwind, *All in Line: An Introduction to the Rolfing Method [Alles im Lot. Eine Einführung in die Rolfing-Methode]*, Droemer Knaur, Munich 2003, p. 173: "However, we are not aware of this anticipatory activity. And for this reason, we remain ignorantly trapped in our habits because these anticipatory activities are present in our movement without our being aware of them in the least."

This process of anticipatory movement activity plays out within the breathing process as well. In other words, a large number of muscle activities precede, accompany, or obstruct the activity of the diaphragm and the rib-lifting musculature. Anticipatory muscle activity guarantees or limits the scope of movement within which the changes in volume necessary for breathing can occur. From this viewpoint, the myofascial units connecting the leg to the pelvic area to the back are of greater significance. These are the layers that are responsible for the position of the hip axis in relation to the torso as a whole. All myofascial units that are attached to the ischial ramus are significant for the tendency of the pelvis to tilt.

The tilting of the pelvis has a considerable influence on the breathing space of the abdomen and thorax. As soon as the pelvis tilts in the posterior direction on the hip axis, the back flattens in the lumbar region and lordosis appears to be reduced. In this case, the radiographic image shows a spine running steeply downward with a small lordotic curvature, but a drastic curve between the last lumbar vertebra and the first, uppermost segment of the sacrum. For the retroperitoneal kidney, the supporting pressure of the posterior layer of the peritoneum is reduced and the effects of gravity create the tendency of the kidneys to sink downward, i.e. into ptosis. This sinking motion may extend to all retro- and subperitoneal elements and will also have an effect on the front of the spine. Because there is no prevertebral musculature above the origin of the psoas that could counteract the downward pull, the innermost deep layer of the chest cavity, the large anterior longitudinal band, finally responds by shortening, and a general equilibrium of tension occurs between the pre- and postvertebral layers of the organism. From a surface observation, the deep erectors of the back appear to be the cause of the tension, but in reality the increase in tone of the erector group is merely a compensatory response to insufficient erection of the column of organs in the interior region of the torso.

The room that is available for breathing motion is influenced by the dynamic described above between prevertebral erection and postvertebral tension. The tilting of the pelvis around the hip axis in the posterior or anterior direction necessarily limits the scope of movement of the diaphragm for

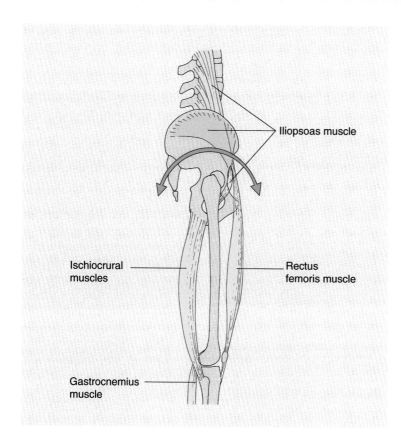

Figure 4.6 Myofascial tensile relationships between the lower extremity and the pelvis.

Iliopsoas muscle

Ischiocrural muscles

Rectus femoris muscle

Gastrocnemius muscle

inhalation. In addition, the room available for breathing motion is dependent upon the upper spatial limits, specifically the spatial limit placed on the ribcage by the pectoral girdle. Because breathing motion is dependent upon the general segmented erection of the body in this fashion, it is necessary to treat the breathing pattern in the context of the overall structure. Here, we place particular emphasis on the tension patterns that occur at the points at which the extremities are connected to the torso:

- in the lower region, the connection between the myofascial units of the musculature of the extremities to the ligaments of the pelvic region
- in the upper region, the shoulder girdle as a bridge between the tension patterns of the arms and ribcage.

If the patient makes an effort to maintain an upright posture, mobilization of the layers that are directly involved in breathing will attain few lasting results. In this case, we must combine the treatment of the breathing pattern with a more global treatment of segmental alignment. In this case, it is important that

- the hip joints have sufficient mobility
- the ligaments of the pelvic region display sufficient elasticity
- the shoulder girdle does not compress the chest cavity too severely
- the organs are able to respond adaptively to the change in volume in the breathing space.

Anatomy of the significant fasciae and membranes of the breathing space

In order for the breathing process to run smoothly, certain conditions of the interior and exterior structure of the torso must be guaranteed:

- The lungs can move or fill only as far as is allowed by the thoracic wall, which is closely adjacent because of the adhesion effect.

- The thoracic wall itself can move only as far as it is allowed space to do so by the generally segmental organization of the erect torso.
- During inhalation, the ribs rise only as far as they are allowed by the intercostal membranes.

Thus, there are exterior limits in the myofascial and membrane structure of the ribcage. In addition, however, there are also interior limits that arise from the fact that individual organs obstruct the motion of the diaphragm. A limitation of breathing motion can arise literally from any fascial or membrane layer or other forms of connective tissue. We can study these limitations using the layered structure of the ribcage. If we wish to reach inward at approximately the level of the fifth rib on the right side of the thorax, we will pass through all fascial and membrane layers that are involved in the active inhalation motion and the passive exhalation motion of the center section of the chest.

The deep fascia is located below the skin and the superficial fatty layer. As the pectoral fascia, it is a continuation of the abdominal fascia. Below the superficial fascia is the myofascial bridge between the external oblique and the serratus anterior. Below this layer, we find the intercostal region with the intercostal musculature and both intercostal membranes, which have different directions in the orientation of their fibers. Farther inward, we find

at individual points the subcostal muscles, each of which has a different path. They are located at the transition between the exterior ribcage structure and the interior layer system of the interior chest wall and exterior pulmonary wall. There are three layers here that are connected to one another by an adhesion effect:

- the endothoracic fascia
- the parietal pleura
- the visceral pleura of the lungs.

Regardless of whether they are located on the outer wall of the ribcage or in the interior cavity, each of these layers can limit normal breathing motion and thus alter the volume patterns of the lungs.

The intercostal membranes are particularly significant. Their elasticity is essential to the movement of the ribs during inhalation. However, this elasticity may extend only to a certain point because the toughness of these membranes is required for the return motion of the ribs in so-called passive breathing. This process of active inhalation and the normally very passive process of exhalation is supported dorsally by the activity of the autonomic musculature of the back, the erector group. In this muscle layer, too, we find a fascial envelope that influences the flexion and extension capacity of the muscles and therefore breathing movement as well. This is the thoracolumbar fascia, which forms an

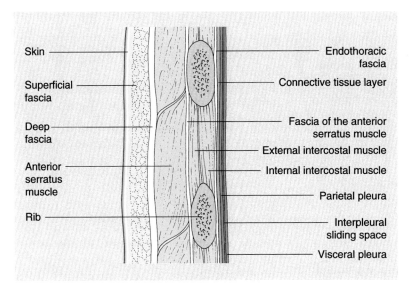

Figure 4.7 Intermediate layers of the thoracic wall.

Skin — Endothoracic fascia

Superficial fascia — Connective tissue layer

Deep fascia — Fascia of the anterior serratus muscle

— External intercostal muscle

— Internal intercostal muscle

Anterior serratus muscle — Parietal pleura

Rib — Interpleural sliding space

— Visceral pleura

osteofibrous canal along with the vertebral arch, dorsal processes, and costal processes. This fascia influences all bending sections of the spine because it is directly connected to the dorsal processes of the thoracic and lumbar spine as well as to the sacrum. In the region of the neck, it continues as the so-called nuchal fascia. Peculiarly, it runs below the trapezius muscle and the rhomboid group in this region. It influences the bending behavior of the spine in this section as well because it is directly connected to the nuchal ligament, which in turn is connected to all of the dorsal processes of the cervical spine.

In addition to the exterior frame structure of the breathing space, the spatial relationship between the visceral cavities of the torso plays an important role. The chest cavity rests above the diaphragm and thus on the organ column of the abdominal and pelvic cavities. The part located inside the peritoneum is dynamic. Owing to constant changes in volume, peristaltic movements, and relatively large changes in the spatial position of the upper abdominal zone, there is a highly movable foundation. In contrast,

the retroperitoneal space is relatively stable. The shear force of the diaphragm has an influence in this region as well; during normal breathing, it moves the kidneys approximately 2 cm. This motion and the muscle activity of the psoas muscle are the dynamic components of the retroperitoneal space. Because they take place without large changes in volume, there is greater stability in this region than in the intraperitoneal space.

The diaphragm forms the foundation of the chest cavity, which is supported by organs. It is surrounded by an elastic membrane on both sides. In addition, a fluid sliding layer, known as the serosa, is located in the regions in which the strongest muscle activity occurs, i.e. on the sides. This serous surrounding layer, which guarantees sliding ability, is not present at the connection point to the liver (area nuda) or in the region of the central tendon.

Conditions are similar for the organs in the peritoneal space. In addition to their own surrounding layer of connective tissue, these organs also have a serous layer that allows sliding during breathing

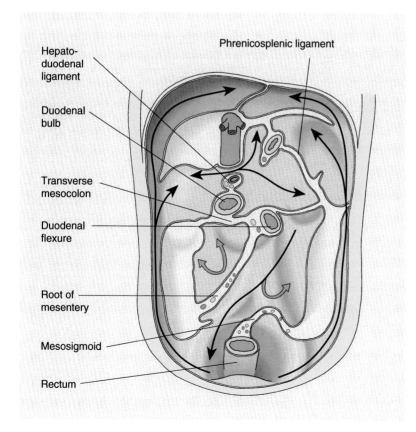

Phrenicosplenic ligament

Hepato-
duodenal
ligament

Duodenal
bulb

Transverse
mesocolon

Duodenal
flexure

Root of
mesentery

Mesosigmoid

Rectum

Figure 4.8 Drainage paths for peritoneal fluid in the abdominal cavity (according to von Lanz/Wachsmuth).

movement. Between the organs, there are actual niches in which the peritoneal fluid can collect and there are gaps inside which the serosa is distributed in certain directions.

> Mobilization techniques for the organs of the upper abdomen, the stomach, the liver, and also for the duodenum and the sections of the colon located farther below, have a particularly lasting effect if the therapist also takes into account the direction of flow of the serous fluid. The mobilization of the organ then simultaneously brings about an improved distribution of the sliding fluid.

The diaphragm changes its shape and position constantly depending upon the position of the body. When sitting, it is somewhat lower than when supine, and when standing it sinks somewhat farther. However, the position of the diaphragm changes even when a person bends to the side, stands overly upright, or sits with a slouch. Therefore, while it is supported from inside by the organ column, it is constantly under the influence of the exterior musculoskeletal system. In this sense, all exterior and interior form-shaping forces are united in the region of the diaphragm. It is precisely for this reason that it seems reasonable to me that the layers adjacent to the diaphragm, i.e. the coatings and ligaments of the organs and the myofascial and membrane frames that surround the diaphragm on the outside, should be treated simultaneously.

I mentioned at the outset that literally all fascial and membrane layers of the organism have significance for the breathing process. To a certain extent, the fasciae located at the transition between the torso and the extremities play a role too.

This is particularly true for the connection between the chest cavity, the pectoral girdle, and the upper extremity. In this region, it is the fascial layers especially that lose their mobility in the course of a lifetime, consisting as they do of a denser material with a higher proportion of collagen fibers relative to the elastin elements. Externally and laterally, this is the fascial boundary between the latissimus dorsi muscle and serratus anterior. In the deep, retrosternal layer, this is especially the transverse thoracis

muscle. It is obvious that the exterior and interior layers are equally important for the development of breathing motion. Therefore, it is worth either using techniques that affect such deep layers and thereby influence the exterior form as well or using techniques that treat the exterior form in such a way that it mobilizes the inner layers as well.

Such a process will prove its value at the upper pole of the breathing mechanism, in the region of the scalene group. In this section of the body, multiple layers of connective tissue overlap. Here, we find extensive fascial layers covering the upper back and shoulder area, layers whose tension patterns mirror a person's dominant emotional habits. However, we also find small myofascial elements such as the subclavius muscle and the minor scalene muscle, which is sometimes missing.

It is not possible to assign a definite emotional meaning to these elements. In any event, they play an important role in securing the breathing mechanism in the upper chest cavity. It is only possible for them to fulfill this role just above and below the clavicle—an area which is so important for the ventilation of the upper lung—if their surrounding fascial layer is elastic enough to allow the lungs to expand here. These layers, which are very significant for breathing motion, have another important duty to perform: they safely channel the nerves and blood vessels between the chest cavity and neck, provided they are subjected to normal tension.

Examination of breathing motion

The most important layers for the breathing process run in the interior of both large visceral cavities and therefore it is possible to access them only to a limited extent through direct touch palpation. The clearest observation of the status of the fasciae may be made by observing the movement behavior of individual components relative to one another, for example, the sliding behavior of the organs relative to one another, as Jean-Pierre Barral has described with his concept of organ mobility (see Chapter 6), or by comparing the sliding behavior of bones, organs, and muscles. We can then clearly determine the fascial and membrane function using the deviation from the norm of the spatial relationships of the individual elements to one another.

For practical examination of breathing motion, the regions in which the various components overlap spatially are significant. This includes the sections in which the visceral cavities meet: the transition between the abdominal and chest cavities and the transition between the chest cavity and the neck region. It is also helpful to include the lower pelvic region and the cranium in the examination with simple tests in order to also take into account the segments of the body that participate in the movement of the diaphragm only in the form of indirect transmission of pressure over large distances.

Evaluation of the transition between the abdominal cavity and thorax

Patient   Seated.

Therapist   Seated behind the patient.

Contact   With both hands: the thumb, index, and middle fingers touch the lower ribs, the ring finger and little finger are in contact with the tissue below the costal arch. Make broad contact with the palm, including the ball of the thumb.

Action   While maintaining a relaxed contact on both sides, the therapist's hands mold closely to the shape of the torso without exerting excessive pressure. It is important for the therapist to sit upright without being tense and to have both feet in firm contact with the floor. Initially the therapist senses the global shearing motion on both sides.

In normal cases it can be felt that:

- The ribs on both sides rise almost identically.
- The ribs perform a rotational motion in the direction of the connection to the vertebral body.
- The intercostal space widens while the spatial curves of the liver and stomach, running opposite one another downward and medially, become perceptible.

At the beginning, precise sensing is required to be able to detect the differences in direction of various components within the general change in volume.

If a smaller increase in volume is evident on one side it reveals a limitation in the movement between the elements of the body under the palpating hand.

In a second observational step, we now concentrate on the spatial, three-dimensional manifestation of this limitation of movement:

- Does the exterior structure appear to be the limitation or is it the deeper layers that are unable to expand?
- Does a characteristic shear motion occur in the direction of the navel due to the tilting behavior of the stomach and/or liver in the direction of the navel?
- Or is the space for intercostal movement limited?

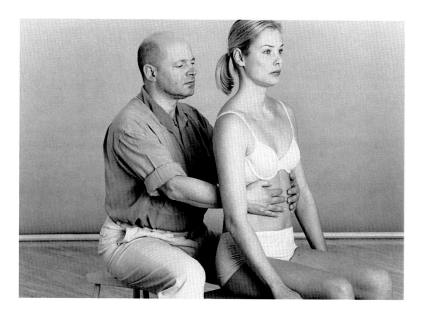

Figure 4.9   Evaluation of the transition between the abdominal cavity and the thorax.

Once the movement of an organ has been limited over an extended period of time, its reduced movement will also be reflected in the surrounding fascial structure of the thorax. This may be an insignificant compensation or a second significant fixation that can considerably influence the fascial network and thus may lead to an exterior fixation of the organ. Then the organ will retain only some of its mobility, even if we have precisely mobilized it, because the scope of movement has been limited from the outside.

Depending on our findings from the test, we must then choose between various treatment steps:

- mobilization of the organ
- mobilization of the intercostal membrane and activation of the fascial layers of the intercostal musculature.
- combined, simultaneous mobilization of the organ with the global fascial framework of the perimeter of the thorax.

In using the last combined technique, it is helpful to perform an additional test in order to precisely determine the fascial connection between the interior and exterior structure of the thorax.

Evaluation of the connection between interior and exterior structure

Patient   Supine, both legs flexed.

Therapist   Sitting next to the side to be evaluated.

Contact   One hand is positioned similarly to the test described above and the other hand is supporting the lumbodorsal transition from below by adapting to the present form.

Action   While the lower hand holds the shape of the back in a slightly flexible yet firm manner, we use the upper hand to place rather more weight on the front of the body. Both hands should exert a small enough amount of force that breathing movement is not limited. It is as if we were holding the exterior fascial structure of the breathing space between our two palms and observing all of the layers running between the interior of the ribs and the stomach or liver in their sliding behavior. The essential step is now to direct our perception to the spatial changes between our two hands and localize the deep layer on the inner edge of the thorax.

This test lends itself to projections in the form of preconceived expectations. The first steps of the test described above are directed at clearly tangible (perceptible) elements that can be directly palpated. In the additional test, we direct our attention to elements with which we are only able to come into contact indirectly, by way of several intermediate layers. This test is a precise detection of the sliding behavior between the parietal pleura, visceral pleura, parietal peritoneum, and visceral peritoneum. The layers we wish to observe fit together in a very tight space and may be best observed if we passively alter the overall shape of the lower part of the thorax by gently lifting it from behind so that we can, so to speak, observe the sliding on the front interior wall of the thorax using a "touch microscope" while the patient's breathing motion continues undisturbed.

Additional test: differentiated evaluation of the transition between the interior and exterior structure with flexible pressure on the costal arch

Patient   Supine, legs flexed.

Therapist   Standing.

Contact   One hand supports the arch of the back and the other hand is adapted to the arch of the lower front side of the thorax.

Action   While the lower hand provides mild resistance, the upper hand provides successive, light pressure in the direction of the front of the spine so that the ribcage yields and then releases gradually, as if in a slow-motion recoil technique. It is now possible:

- to compare the elasticity of the intercostal membranes
- to localize precisely the defective mobility of individual ribs
- to evaluate the volume space in the lower ribcage in relation to the interior movement of the organs.

Once we have compressed the patient's ribcage between both hands for several breathing cycles, we can precisely localize present or defective sliding on the inner wall of the thorax.

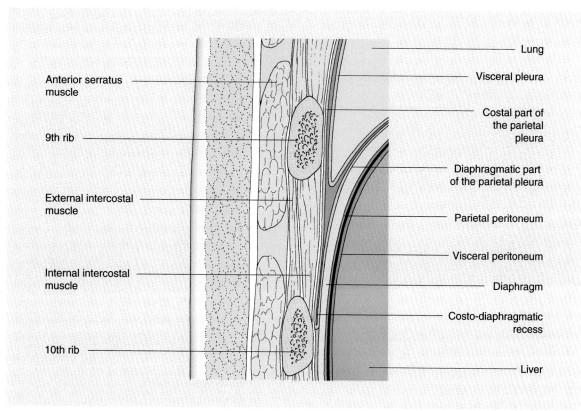

Figure 4.10   Layers of the thoracic wall in the region of the overlapping of the visceral pleura, diaphragm, and liver.

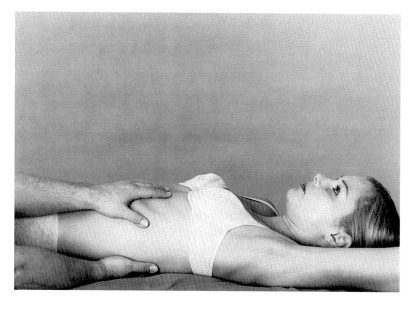

Figure 4.11   Evaluation of the connection between the interior and exterior structure.

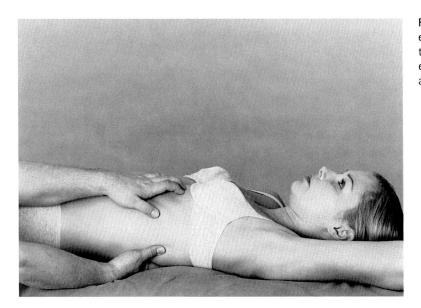

Figure 4.12   Differentiated evaluation of the transition between the interior and exterior structure: elastic pressure against the costal arch.

It is possible to perform this test with various intensities of pressure and slight variations in the vector of pressure. The fundamental rule is: the more voluminous the thorax is in the sagittal plane, the steeper the appropriate vector of pressure. The test is contraindicated or should be used with the greatest caution if entire groups of ribs have been concavely deformed (scoliosis) or if rib fractures are present that have not completely healed.

Evaluation of the transition between the upper chest cavity and the neck region in the sagittal plane

Patient   Seated.

Therapist   Standing next to the patient.

Contact   With the thumb and index finger on the posterior side below the second rib, parallel to the course of the bone shape, but with the thumb and index finger on the anterior side analogously positioned below under both clavicles parallel to the course of the bone shape.

Action   Both supporting hands create contact with the layers of tissue between the bony structures: on the posterior side, with the layers between the second and third rib and, on the anterior side, with the layers between the clavicle and the first rib, i.e. in the region of the subclavius muscle and the layers connected to it.

While the patient breathes normally, we now observe and sense how the breathing process manifests as a change in volume on the anterior and posterior sides. In a normal case, the impression arises on the posterior side that the second pair of ribs is sinking slightly while the adjacent vertebral bodies become erect. However, this movement can be discerned only if there is a balanced coordination between the musculature of the ribcage and pectoral girdle and the patient's shoulders are not pulled upward during inhalation. The normal movement in the region of the upper ribs requires the simultaneous physiological movement of the shoulders.

In a normal case, we will feel on the front that the first rib is gently moving our examining hand upward against the clavicles.

In order to comprehensively evaluate the condition of the fascial system in the upper chest cavity, we should now compare the shear movement in the anterior portion with the tangible movement in the posterior section and, at the same time, turn our attention to any differences on the sides before we move on to a detailed analysis of the deep layers in this region.

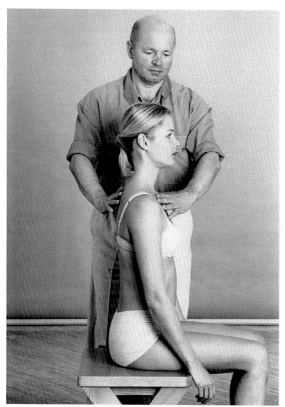

Figure 4.13   Evaluation of the transition between the upper chest cavity and the neck area in the sagittal plane.

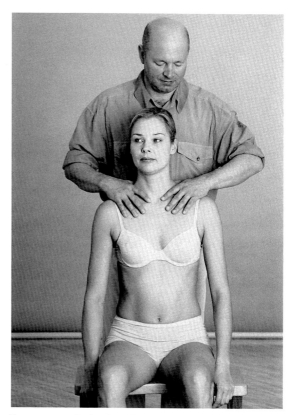

Figure 4.14   Evaluation of the deep layers from the anterior side.

Additional test: evaluation of the deep layers
from the anterior side

Patient   Seated.

Therapist   Standing behind the patient.

Contact   With the thumbs on the posterior side over the first rib, with the index fingers on the anterior side on the medial sections of the pleura cupulas, with the remaining fingers of both hands under the clavicles.

Action   While the thumbs serve as fixed points from the posterior side, the fingers compare the mobility of both pleural cupulas and the connection between the two clavicles and the first rib (subclavius muscle).

Evaluation of breathing movement in the lower pelvic region

Patient   Supine, legs outstretched, arms resting on either side of the torso.

Therapist   Seated to the side at the level of the patient's hips.

Contact   One hand supports the sacrum from the posterior side while the second hand rests superior to the joint of the pubic bone.

In women, we must keep in mind that the uterus has a different position when the bladder or descending colon is full. In men, a reduction in breathing movement in this region provides information regarding the pressure conditions acting on the prostate in the lower pelvis. The purpose of this test is to ascertain the mobility of the intraperitoneal elements in relation to that of the extraperitoneal elements.

Action   The therapist supports the sacrum with one hand and, with the other hand, comes into

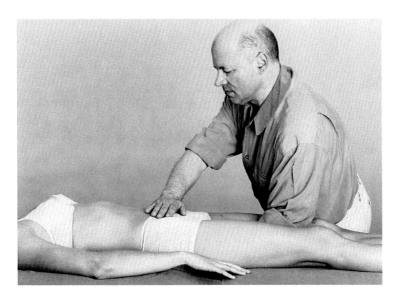

Figure 4.15   Examination of breathing motion in the lower pelvic region.

contact with the tissue layers above the pubic bone. In a normal case, the base of the sacrum will move dorsally during inhalation and lumbar lordosis will be reduced, while the elements inside and outside the peritoneum slide opposite one another. We can now ascertain whether the limitation of movement is primarily manifest in the back or the anterior chamber of the pelvis and then select our treatment strategy depending on what we find.

Evaluation of breathing movement in the retroperitoneal area

Patient   Lying on one side.

Therapist   Seated to the side at the level of the hips.

Contact   With the thumb below the twelfth rib.

Action   The therapist's thumb reaches parallel to the twelfth rib in the direction of the lower boundary of the kidneys until the therapist is able to feel the shear effect of breathing motion. If the kidney is too low or clearly limited in its movement, the shear is not easy to detect during inhalation. In any event, a comparison should be made between the two sides.

Evaluation of the transmission of breathing motion into the cranium

Patient   Supine, legs outstretched, arms resting on either side of the torso.

Therapist   Seated near the head.

Contact   With both palms in the region of the parietal bone.

Action   Breathing motion can only become discernible in the cranium if an elastic effect is allowed by the forces acting on the cranium. If the falx of the cerebrum overall is subjected to strong tensile force between the base of the skull and the frontal bone, this sort of elastic effect cannot occur. It is essential for this test to exercise slightly elastic pressure on both sides from the lateral direction in order to ascertain whether the cranium springs back. Subsequently, with gentle contact, the therapist's attention is then directed toward whether the breathing motion can be felt in the cranium.

Treatment of the fascial network of the respiratory area

Treatment of the deep fascia and intercostal membranes

Patient   Supine, both legs flexed.

Therapist   Standing at the level of the patient's hips.

Contact   From behind with a flat hand in the region of the middle thoracolumbar fascia, from

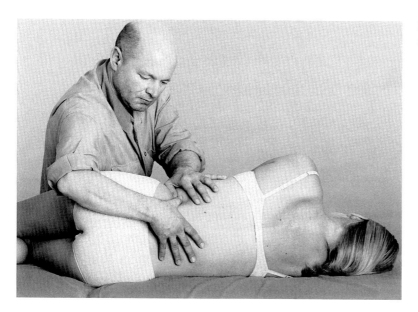

Figure 4.16   Evaluation of breathing motion in the retroperitoneal area.

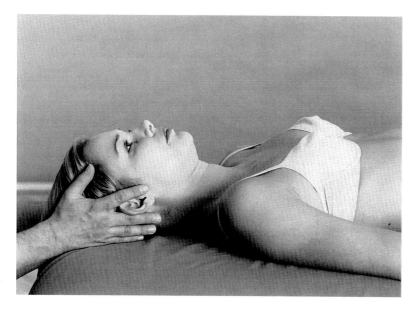

Figure 4.17   Evaluation of the transmission of breathing motion into the cranium.

the front with a flat hand directly at the transition between the abdominal and chest cavities with the fingertips between the region of the middle ribs.

Action   The therapist gently supports the curvature of the back with a flat hand from behind. The therapist's palm stays in contact with the superficial and deep layers of the back in that the weight of the therapist's hand is placed on the table and the palm is adapted as precisely as possible to the curvature of the back. The therapist's other hand maintains a flat contact with the lower ribs and, at the same time, its fingertips reach through the subcutaneous fat to the deep fascia in order to exert a stretching impulse in a slightly cranial and medial direction. If restrictions of movement can be found in the deeper intercostal region when examining the chest area, the pressure being exerted by the fingertips should be directed somewhat more steeply inward. The steeper the direct pressure is

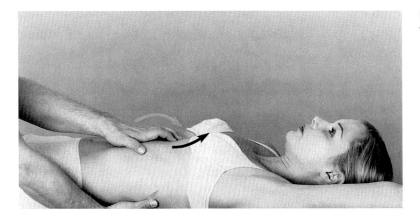

Figure 4.18 Treatment of the deep fascia and intercostal membranes.

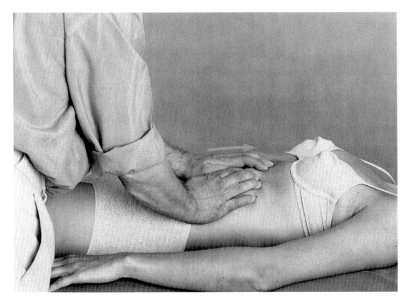

Figure 4.19 Treatment of the upper section of the fascia of the rectus abdominis.

exerted, the more interior its effect reaches. In this manner, it is possible to reach the intercostal and subcostal regions.

It is important that both of the therapist's palms remain "listening" while the fingertips are active. "Listening" is very important because we should only stretch the surface sufficiently that we can track the inner elements of the chest cavity. Support in the dorsal region plays an essential role for the efficiency of this technique. The more strongly the pressure is exerted on the anterior side, the firmer the support from the dorsal direction should be.

Treatment of the upper section of the fascia of the rectus abdominis

Patient   Supine, both legs flexed.

Therapist   Standing next to the treatment table approximately at the level of the patient's hips.

Contact   With the flat front of the phalanges of both hands on the level of the intersection of tendons at the rectus abdominis muscle.

Action   In this technique as well, the therapist's palms are "listening." The therapist's phalanges reach through the superficial layer, through the abdominal part of the pectoralis major and gently make contact with the deeper layers of the rectus

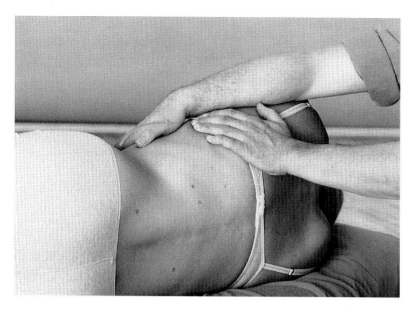

Figure 4.20   Treatment of the fascial boundary between the serratus anterior and the oblique abdominal muscle.

abdominis. With the more lateral hand, the therapist gives a slight push in the cranial and medial direction toward the sternum. With the hand that was applied medially, the therapist applies a slight, direct, stretching effect in the cranial direction. Both hands move slightly in the anterior direction, while the hand applied farther outward moves diagonally toward the hand applied in the middle region. With some skill, it is possible to use this compression to reach the posterior section of the sheath of the rectus as well.

Treatment of the fascial boundary between the serratus anterior and the oblique abdominal muscle

Patient   Lying on one side, knee slightly flexed.

Therapist   Sitting next to the treatment table at the level of the chest cavity.

Contact   Both hands are in flat contact, with a somewhat firmer contact through the front phalanges.

Action   The therapist adapts both hands as precisely as possible to the exterior shape of the ribcage. While maintaining the surface contact with both hands, one hand exercises a tensional force on the fascia of the oblique abdominal muscle in the direction of the course of the muscle fibers. At the same time, the other hand pushes the serratus anterior in the direction of the oblique abdominal muscle. In the region of the serratus muscle, contact is parallel to the course of the muscle fibers. Thus, the two muscles are moved toward each other in such a way that they are pushing against each other somewhat at their point of overlap. While applying somewhat more pressure along the arc of the ribs of the chest cavity, both of the therapist's hands are moved toward one another and cause a direct stretching of the fascial layers of both muscles mentioned above.

If this technique is used on the left side of the body, it may be used in a somewhat modified manner for treatment restrictions of mobility of the spleen. For this purpose, it is necessary to limit contact with the muscular fasciae by the fingertips and work solely with the flat palm of the hand. Naturally, the limitation of movement of the superficial musculature and fascial layer may also be treated at the same time as deeper organ structures. In this case, the active use of the fingertips acts on the muscular fascia while the subtly applied pressure of both palms is directed deeper and influences the mobility of the spleen.

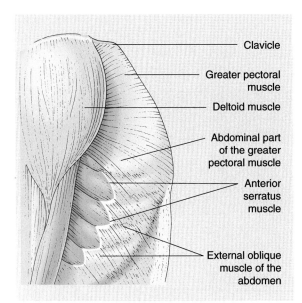

Clavicle

Greater pectoral muscle

Deltoid muscle

Abdominal part of the greater pectoral muscle

Anterior serratus muscle

External oblique muscle of the abdomen

Figure 4.21 Myofascial connection between the serratus anterior and the oblique abdominal muscle.

Treatment of the sternoclavicular connection

Patient   Supine, legs flexed.

Therapist   Sitting at the level of the patient's shoulders.

Contact   With one hand from the posterior direction between the first and second ribs, with the other hand parallel to the clavicle in the direction of the sternoclavicular joint.

Action   The therapist supports the scapula from below and reaches with the fingers precisely between the first and second ribs. With the other hand, the therapist reaches toward the sternoclavicular joint parallel to the clavicle, maintaining light contact with the clavicle itself so that it can be easily compressed into the joint connection. The therapist now gradually intensifies contact with this hand so that it is exerting a shearing force on the joint. The therapist then intensifies the pressure from the posterior and anterior directions as if to move the contact surfaces of both hands toward one another. The contact from the posterior direction acts as a wedge between the first and second ribs. With the hand applied on the anterior side, the therapist now intensifies the pressure until a

discernible countertension builds up next to the sternoclavicular joint, which the therapist follows until the sternoclavicular connection opens into a larger movement pattern.

> To a certain extent, the technique described above is similar to the treatment technique shown in the section on the pectoral girdle (see section 4.3) for the layers of the subclavius muscle. In contrast to the subclavius technique, however, it acts in a far more direct manner on the inner joint connection of the sternoclavicular joint, in particular on the ligaments stabilizing the joint. In the case of an actual joint fixation, it is advisable to use the hand applied on the anterior side to surround the clavicle and guide it into the joint capsule. With subsequent "listening," following the directional pulls of tendon tension, it is possible to act precisely on the joint itself.

Treatment of the posterior section of the scalene fascia

Patient   Supine, both legs flexed.

Therapist   Standing at the head of the treatment table.

Contact   Supporting the head from the posterior direction with one hand and with the other hand coming from the lateral direction toward the fascia of the posterior scalene muscle.

Action   Here, it is important for both of the patient's legs to be flexed because this creates a push in the cranial direction and the neck is lengthened from its connection to the ribcage. The therapist lifts the occiput slightly and, at the same time, brings the entire neck region into a slight rotation and sideways bend. At the same moment, the therapist's other hand reaches in the direction of the posterior scalene muscle. The target is the deep section of the lateral portions of the lamina of the neck. The rotation and sideways tilt of the neck is necessary in order to keep all of the superficial muscular elements completely relaxed. Only in this way can

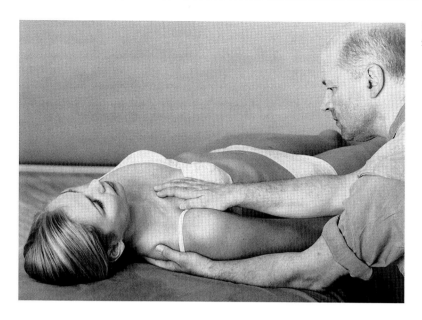

Figure 4.22 Treatment of the sternoclavicular connection.

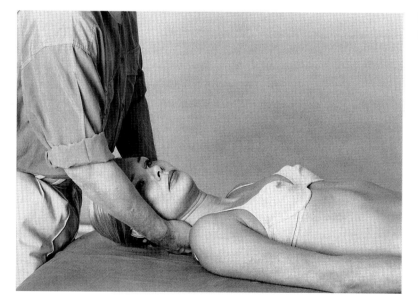

Figure 4.23 Treatment of the posterior section of the scalene fascia.

contact be produced in the direction of the scalene fascia. As soon as the therapist is able to detect breathing motion of the scalene group at this point, the therapist intensifies the contact in the direction of the transverse processes of the cervical spine. At this moment, the contact point should not slide. Rather, it is necessary to hold the contact like an elastic hook. In a second step, it is now necessary to move the head a little farther in its sideways curve and rotation while an intense pull in the mediocranial direction is exerted on the contact point of the posterior scalene muscle. The pull should be parallel to the direction of the muscle fibers of the scalene muscle and avail itself of only a minimal sliding motion. By changing the position of the head, it is possible to reach different layers.

Treatment of pleural adhesions in the upper chest cavity

After the treatment of the upper part of the scalene musculature, it is important to examine the onset region at the upper ribs more precisely, in particular to examine the parietal pleura for any adhesions that may be present. The treatment of a pleural adhesion is an essential supplement to the treatment of the scalene.

Patient   Supine, both legs flexed.

Therapist   Standing at the level of the patient's lower ribs.

Contact   Supporting the back from the posterior side with one hand, while at the same time subtly contacting the anterior side with the palm of the other hand.

Action   The therapist takes the ribcage in both hands from a posterior and lateral direction. It is important for this technique that the therapist's supporting hand coming from the posterior and lateral direction reflects not the exterior shape of the structure of the chest wall, but rather the inner structure. For this purpose, it is necessary to compress the entire rib structure somewhat at the lateral–posterior transition, specifically at the precise height at which the pleural adhesion may be found from the anterior direction. Thus, we follow the effect of the intake of air into the lungs and, in this manner, somewhat alter the sliding behavior of the interior layers of the chest cavity. At the same time, our hand applied on the anterior side moves along precisely in the direction of a pull effect occurring inward. We follow the movement until it comes to a stop. At that moment, we break off contact.

In this technique, we use contact from the posterior direction as a fixed point and follow from the anterior direction while "listening." In so doing, we try to maintain contact as precisely as possible with the pleural fixation. This technique can be varied very effectively if

we select the fixed point directly from the front. In this case, the subtle pressure of our hand falls precisely at the point of the limitation of movement. While we are now holding the limitation of movement from the front side, we rotate the upper chest cavity around the vertical axis of the upper lungs. This rotation should only be conducted in minimal steps. If we apply this technique carefully, we will be able to influence the sliding behavior of the major intermediate layers of the upper chest cavity relative to one another and, in so doing, reduce the extent of the pleural adhesion.

Treatment of the sternum and the transversus thoracic muscle

Patient   Prone.

Therapist   Seated at the head.

Contact   With the fingers of both hands directly on the sternum.

Action   In order to guarantee the efficacy of this technique, it is necessary for the patient to transfer the entire weight of the thorax onto the treatment table while relaxing as much as possible. The therapist's fingertips now feel through the generally very thin subcutaneous layer in the region of the sternum in the direction of the periosteum of the sternum. The therapist asks the patient to allow the weight of the upper body to sink somewhat more against the contact of the therapist's fingers. In so doing, the sternum moves in the anterior direction. With the fingers of both hands, the therapist now intensifies the contact, paying attention to whether parts of the bones in individual areas appear to be denser or less elastic. It is precisely at these points that the therapist intensifies the pressure, as if to reach inward through the sternum into the retrosternal cavity. If the therapist's hands are removed from one another, the therapist follows this movement and is therefore able to influence intraosseus tensions of the sternum. In a subsequent step, the therapist's entire attention is focused on whether the hands are being pulled inward at individual sections of the

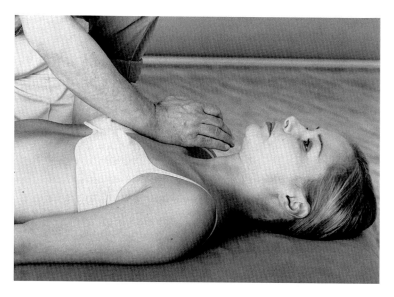

Figure 4.24   Treatment of pleural adhesions in the upper chest cavity.

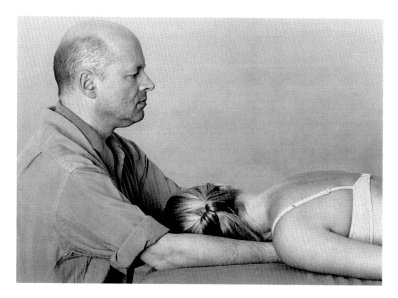

Figure 4.25   Treatment of the sternum and the transversus thoracis muscle.

sternum. The therapist follows the drawing effect inward and thus guides the sternum in the direction of the retrosternal organs. In this manner, a change occurs in the tone pattern of the transversus thoracis muscle, which is autonomically controlled to a large extent. As soon as the therapist feels a strong counterpressure beginning to build up behind the sternum, the quality of the touch should be intensified again and finally be released once a response of the autonomic nervous system is manifested by a deep, tension-releasing breath by the patient.

This technique is also particularly effective in the case of organ fixations. The myofascial layers located directly behind the sternum are directly connected to the interpleural space and ligament attachment of the heart. This technique shows that parietal and visceral structures in the thoracic region are closely connected and that it is reasonable to treat them simultaneously.

Specific influence on the interpleural space

Patient   Supine, legs extended.

Therapist   Standing at the level of the abdominal cavity.

Contact   From the posterior side approximately at the level of the tenth thoracic vertebra with the palm and from the anterior side approximately in the middle of the sternum.

Action   The therapist provides support from the posterior direction with a flat palm at the level of the tenth thoracic vertebra, exerting contact not against the spinous processes but rather on both sides on the strands of muscle next to the spine. The other hand contacts the front of the sternum from the anterior direction, initially using only the weight of the forearm and the hand. In this manner, the interior elasticity of the sternum can be evaluated, as well as the manner in which it is connected to the ribs. As soon as the therapist's tactile attention has been directed somewhat farther inward, he or she receives information about the mobility of the interpleural space and the pericardium. In so doing, it is important for the contact to be applied sufficiently high above the diaphragm to avoid the tensile effect of the central tendon of the diaphragm. The therapist now intensifies the contact so that the touch is having an indirect effect behind the sternum. The quality of the touch remains extremely subtle, even when the pressure applied is increased slightly. Only in this manner is it possible to feel if the sliding behavior of the serous layers is reduced. The boundary between diagnosis and therapy in this area is fluid. Technically, it is important for the support from the posterior direction not to be stiff, but still to be sustained enough that the hand acting from the anterior direction is not able to push the organ cavity as a whole too far in the posterior direction. If a fixation exists in the region of the interpleural space or the pericardium, the hand will make minimal tilting or rotational movements. The anterior hand of the therapist follows this movement until the retrosternal space responds with a slight expansion. At this moment, the therapist removes the anterior hand and only then allows the hand providing support in the posterior direction to follow.

In the case of a restriction of movement that has existed for a long time, the interior shape of the ribcage will have changed during this time. Thus, the restriction of movement is present not only in the membrane layers directly related to organs but also in the muscular and membrane structure of the intercostal region. In this case, it is wise first to treat the sternum and transversus thoracis muscle globally, followed by the subtle correction of the structures related to the organs. If the restrictions of movement have occurred in the interior of the chest cavity as a result of a global posture pattern, it is helpful for the chest cavity to be pretreated as in the following techniques.

Treatment of the thoracocervical transition

Patient   Sitting upright on a stool.

Therapist   Sitting on a footstool in front of the patient.

Contact   With the base and surface of the thumb below both clavicles.

Action   For this treatment technique, it is important for the patient's feet to have good contact with the floor and for the abdominal wall to be completely relaxed. The patient should imagine his or her clavicle joint sinking very slightly while the ischial bones expand downward so that the pelvis tilts slightly in the anterior direction around the hip axis. The patient keeps the sternum relatively high and leans against the therapist's two hands, which are primarily maintaining contact below the clavicles with the base of the thumb and the thumbs. The therapist structures this contact in such a way that the effect of the touch expands into the region of the upper chest cavity. In general, the endothoracic fascia is very thin, but it thickens in this upper region and functions in conjunction with the scalene fascia as a suspending connection of the upper pleural cupulas. The goal of our technique is to move this suspending connection in the cranial direction, toward its origin, while the sternum literally hangs vertically below the clavicle between our contact points. As an

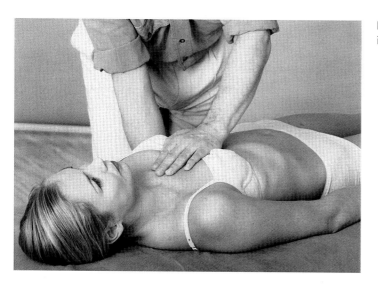

Figure 4.26 Specific influence on the interpleural space.

additional treatment step, the therapist asks the patient to hold the neck upright while keeping the pectoral girdle relaxed. In this manner, we achieve a direct influence on the space between the lower cervical spine, the pectoral girdle, and the upper chest cavity, which is so important for respiration.

> A normal low level of asymmetry between the two sides of the upper sternum will always be discernible. However, if there are obvious restrictions of movement, it is always wise to check whether there has been previous trauma. In this case, it is better initially to treat the affected side while the patient is lying down and then to follow up with the treatment in the sitting position as an "integrative post-treatment."

Treatment of the myofascial structures between the upper chest cavity and the upper section of the back

Patient Sitting on a stool.

Therapist Standing next to the patient.

Contact One palm rests at the level of the third thoracic vertebra from a posterior direction while the other hand rests on both sides below the clavicle from the anterior direction.

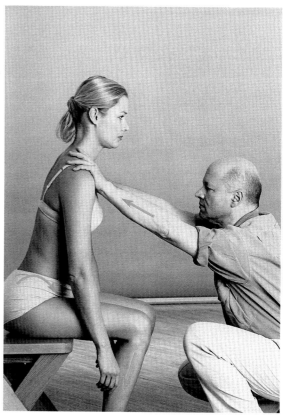

Figure 4.27 Treatment of the thoracocervical transition.

Action The patient first tilts the pelvis slightly in the anterior direction and then leans forward somewhat with the entire torso while keeping the head upright. The therapist receives the

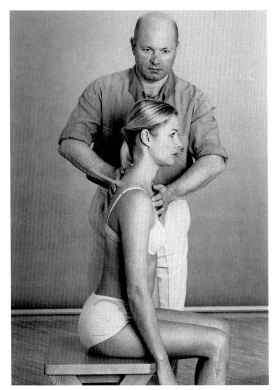

Figure 4.28 Treatment of the myofascial structures between the upper chest cavity and the upper section of the back.

patient's body weight with the hand applied from the anterior direction and, at the same time, applies pressure from the posterior direction to the myofascial layers on both sides of the spine. The pressure from both hands is maintained as if the therapist were moving them toward one another. The therapist asks the patient to intensify the contact between the feet and the floor so that the entire torso becomes somewhat more erect by means of an interior push. While this is occurring, the therapist maintains contact firmly with both hands so that the deep interior layers of the thoracocervical transition are pushed in the cranial direction between the therapist's hands. In this manner, a drastic stretching effect is mainly achieved by the patient's actions because the relevant layers cannot be reached by the therapist's hands.

Treatment of the myofascial complex of the lateral thorax

Patient Lying on one side with knees flexed.

Therapist Sitting facing the patient's back.

Contact The patient lies on both of the therapist's hands beneath the side to be treated.

Action The therapist allows the forearms to rest on the treatment table and surrounds as much as possible of the lateral portion of the ribs with both palms. In so doing, it is important that the therapist's hands be adapted to the shape of the body in such a way that the palms precisely reflect the arch of the ribs. It is crucial that the therapist support the weight of the patient's upper body in such a way that the exterior myofascial layers relax somewhat and the pressure of the therapist's hands is transmitted farther inward in the intercostal region to the interior wall of the thorax and the subcostal layers. As soon as the therapist is able to feel the patient's weight being increasingly transferred onto the therapist's hands, the therapist successively intensifies the pressure with both hands as if to reduce somewhat the sagittal extension of the chest cavity. A pull now becomes discernible that works on the thoracic wall from the interior. It is now important to follow this pull while the rib structure remains compressed with elastic pressure. If the therapist's hands are displaced from one another by a pull that can be felt from the interior, it is important to follow the movement, but still maintain compression of the exterior structure of the ribs. Compression of the exterior rib arch is so important because this is how we can gain influence over the sliding behavior of the parietal pleura in this region. It is in the vicinity of the diaphragm that the parietal pleura has elastic fibers that can respond to the altered sliding behavior.

Treatment of the fascial connection between the chest cavity and the pectoral girdle

Patient Lying on one side with the head supported by a pillow.

Therapist Standing to one side at the head.

Contact The patient's upper arm rests on the forearm of the therapist and is as relaxed as possible; the therapist's fingers make contact with the axillary fascia while the other hand maintains a flat contact at the transition between the chest cavity and upper arm.

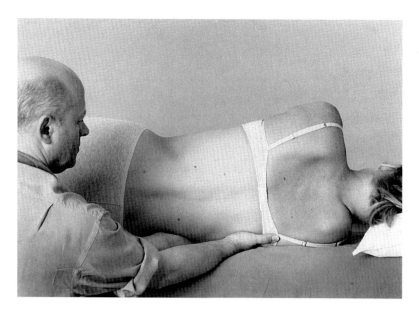

Figure 4.29   Treatment of the myofascial complex of the lateral thorax.

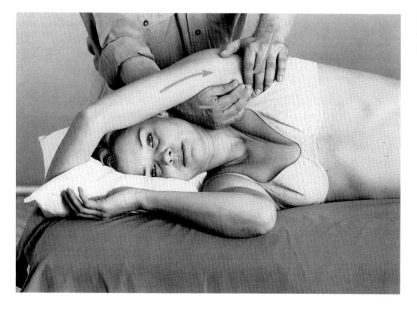

Figure 4.30   Treatment of the fascial connection between the chest cavity and the pectoral girdle.

Action   The patient's arm should be positioned so as not to pull on the joint capsule. The therapist now eases the patient's upper arm into the shoulder joint. The pressure should be sufficient only to allow the deep joint structures to relax somewhat. At the same time, with the other hand, the therapist makes flat contact at the transition between the upper chest cavity and the arm. The therapist keeps this contact elastic but still very firm using the weight of the hand and forearm and now changes the angle at which the patient's upper arm is supported relative to the ribcage. In so doing, it is possible to reach various deep layers of the fascial system, the fascial network, in its three-dimensional structure. The precondition for a lasting effect is that the therapist maintain firm contact at the transition between the chest cavity and the arm and that the patient allow the upper arm to be passively moved.

Treatment techniques for the diaphragm and adjacent membranes

Because we cannot directly touch the diaphragm, we must use an indirect process to treat it. For this reason, the treatment of the diaphragm is also the treatment of the frame surrounding the diaphragm and the treatment of membrane coverings and bands running between the diaphragm and other organs. The exterior frame of movement of the diaphragm is limited by the bone, muscle, and membrane structure of the ribcage. Its interior frame of movement is limited by the relative movability of the organs located below the diaphragm, in particular the liver and stomach. Here, it is important to keep in mind that the liver is firmly connected to the diaphragm in the region of the so-called area nuda.

Treatment of the upper diaphragm boundary

Before using this technique, it is necessary to use the test process described to ascertain which cupula of the diaphragm is the more restricted in its movement. The technique should be used on this side first.

Patient   Supine, both legs extended.

Therapist   Standing somewhat below the boundary of the diaphragm.

Contact   With the palm of one hand and the back of the other hand in the region of the upper diaphragm cupula.

Action   The therapist creates contact with the thoracic wall so that the palm and fingers are adapted to the arch of the ribcage. With the palm and back of the other hand, the therapist applies gradually increasing pressure in the direction of the sternum as if to turn one half of the thorax in toward the sternum or in toward the connection with the sternum. With some care, the therapist will be able to follow how a countermotion occurs on the interior wall of the ribcage as if cylinders inserted into one another were beginning to turn in opposite directions. The therapist now maintains the pressure in the direction of the sternum until the countermotions discernible from the deep layers come to a stop. At this moment, the therapist allows the pressure contact to become weaker and follows the rebounding movement of the structure of the ribcage in the lateral direction. In principle, this is a very slow application of the recoil principle. However, it is indispensable for the desired effect that we avoid a recoil effect that snaps back and follow the ribcage in all of its changes of direction into a larger expansion in the lateral direction.

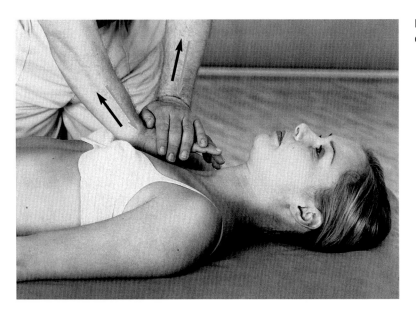

Figure 4.31   Treatment of the upper diaphragm boundary.

Treatment of the lower diaphragm boundary

Patient Supine.

Therapist Sitting at the level of the patient's hips.

Contact One hand supports the lowermost region of the ribcage from the posterior direction while the other hand produces a flat contact at the same level between the lateral section and the front of the ribcage.

Action The therapist raises the lower thoracic region slightly such that the lordotic arch of the lumbar spine continues minimally in the lower region of the thoracic spine. At the same time, the therapist's other hand exerts compression from the lateral direction. The therapist applies pressure diagonally through the lower chest cavity in the direction of the twelfth thoracic vertebra, more specifically in the direction of the front of the anterior side of this vertebra.

Here, we are exploiting the fact that the abdominal organs are somewhat higher in relation to the diaphragm when the body is lying down and the diaphragm itself also appears to have been displaced somewhat in the cranial direction. In other words, we use the framework of the lower thorax to intensify the tendency followed by the diaphragm in the lower chest cavity when lying down. This process may last for several breaths. We intensify the elastic pressure until a strong movement is evident during inhalation. At this moment, we first reduce contact on the front side and then also on the back side. Here as well, we are avoiding the recoil effect so that, during the release, we can follow the various directions of movement step by step that manifest on the thoracic wall.

The hand providing support from the posterior direction acts as a slightly elastic fixed point while the hand applied in front can change the direction of pressure several times during this process. Caution is necessary in the case of poorly healed rib fractures or scoliosis, in particular of ribs that are curved inward in the anterior region on the side to be treated. This technique may be applied on both sides of the thorax. On the right side, this technique is also suitable for treating restrictions of movement in the region of the coronary ligament and/or the right triangular ligament.

Simultaneous treatment of the diaphragm cupulas

Patient Supine, legs extended.

Therapist Standing at the level of the hip joint.

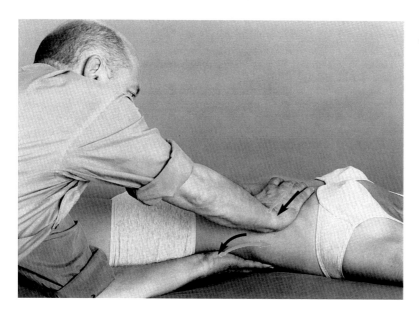

Figure 4.32 Treatment of the lower diaphragm boundary.

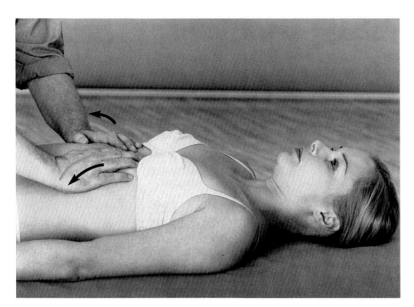

Figure 4.33 Simultaneous treatment of the diaphragm cupulas.

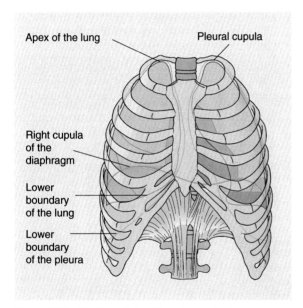

Figure 4.34 Spatial relationship between the lung, pleura, and diaphragm from the anterior direction.

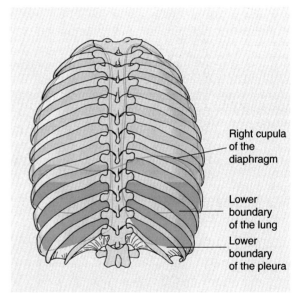

Figure 4.35 Spatial relationship between the lung, pleura, and diaphragm from the posterior direction.

Contact With both hands flat in the region in which the lower portion of the pleura, the diaphragm, and the sheath layers of the liver and/or the peritoneum overlap spatially.

Action The therapist now successively applies somewhat more weight in both hands and, from both sides, exerts diagonal pressure in the direction of the sternum. The therapist gradually compresses both halves of the thorax in this region, taking care that this gradual increase in pressure comes from the therapist's upper body weight shifting into the hands, while avoiding stiffness in the shoulders and elbows. The pressure should continue only until the thorax yields in a slightly elastic manner. If one half of the thorax provides resistance, it is important initially to respect this resistance and, coming from the other side, to press the other half of the thorax against this resistance until it diminishes somewhat. In this technique, it is important that the therapist avoid resistances by varying the direction of pressure. As soon as a strong counter-pressure becomes noticeable, the contact from both hands is slowly released. This release should be fluid and gradual, with the therapist initially avoiding contact with the side where the stronger pressure had build up.

Carefully executed, this technique can influence the exterior structure of the ribcage as well as the interior connections between organs in relation to the diaphragm. In order to reach both areas, it is necessary for the therapist not to slide on the contact areas, but rather to maintain consistent contact with the subcutaneous tissues and deep fascia. It is sometimes helpful to actually anchor the fingertips in the superficial and deep fascia while the palms concentrate on the interior layers of the body with their perception and combine an indirect influence on the organ region with active influence on the surface of the chest cavity.

Treatment of the relationship between the liver and the right cupula of the diaphragm

Patient   Lying on the left side with knees slightly flexed.

Therapist   Standing at the level of the pelvis.

Contact   With the relaxed edge of the hand below the right costal arch and with the other hand flat in the lateral region of the middle and lower ribs.

Action   The therapist initially gently touches the region below the patient's right costal arch with the edge of the right hand. The quality of this touch should be completely free of any penetrating vector. Then the palm of the therapist's other hand creates an elastic contact with the ribcage in the lateral region of the middle and lower ribs. In the next treatment step, the therapist compresses this rib section, precisely toward the patient's navel. In

so doing, the therapist pushes the costal arch somewhat over the edge of the therapist's right hand, which thus moves farther inward and carefully makes contact with the liver. Because the therapist is compressing the exterior structure of the chest cavity in the sagittal direction, the liver can clearly follow its suspension on the coronary ligament and the right triangular ligament. It is as though the therapist, by compressing the chest cavity, pushes the tensional forces originating from the chest cavity into the background for a few moments, thus allowing the therapist's tactile observation of the relationship between the liver and the diaphragm to be more precise. The patient's position on the left side supports the natural movement of the liver during inhalation in the direction of the navel. If this movement cannot be felt in spite of the chest cavity being compressed, this is a clear indication of a restriction. It is best to treat this restriction by continuing to compress the chest cavity from the side and, with the hand below the costal arch, lifting the liver precisely in the direction of the discernible restriction and subsequently releasing it again slowly. Under certain circumstances, the fixation of the liver may be detected precisely in the region of the right triangular ligament. In this case, it is possible for the therapist to increase the efficiency of this technique by moving the hands toward one another precisely in the direction of the course of the fibers of the triangular ligament.

Treatment variation for the relationship between the liver and diaphragm

Patient   Lying on the right side with the knees slightly flexed.

Therapist   Standing at the level of the patient's hips.

Contact   The therapist encloses the patient's right side, with the patient transferring his or her weight precisely at the level of the liver into the therapist's hand. With the ball of the thumb of the other hand, the therapist makes contact with the left costal arch while making contact with the stomach with the palm of the hand.

Action   The therapist's right hand supports the side on which the patient is lying. The therapist makes sure not to apply strong pressure to less elastic ribs so as to allow the exterior layers of the

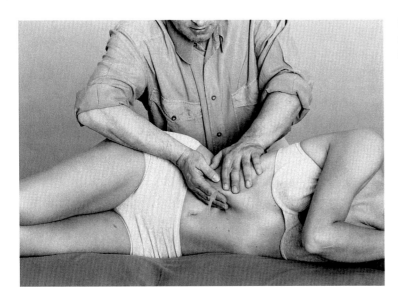

Figure 4.36   Treatment of the relationship between the liver and the right cupula of the diaphragm.

ribcage to relax. In so doing, the quality of the therapist's touch should be such that the density of the tissue structure of the liver can be felt. With the other hand, the therapist now compresses the ribcage so that the connection of the stomach with its ligamentous suspension relaxes somewhat. During this, the therapist feels with the palm of the hand how the pyloric end of the stomach moves somewhat in the direction of the right side of the body. As soon as this movement becomes discernible, the therapist gently lifts the liver against the stomach and, by "listening," follows the stomach as well as the liver until the movement comes to a stop.

This technique is particularly suitable for restrictions between the liver and the diaphragm that have been present for a long time. For example, for restrictions caused by hepatitis that have influenced the mobility of the organ as a whole I am of the opinion that prolonged restrictions of an organ can deform the inner shape of the chest cavity in a very lasting manner. It is possible that the deformations occur due to spasm-like changes of tone in the region of the intercostal or subcostal musculature. The advantage of the technique described above lies in the fact that it not only works for detail fixations, but also treats the global interrelations of space in the lower chest cavity.

Treatment of the stomach in its relationship to the left cupula of the diaphragm

Patient   Resting on the right side with knees slightly flexed.

Therapist   Standing at the level of the patient's costal arch.

Contact   With the flat left hand laterally on the costal arch and with the relaxed edge of the right hand approximately in the region of the sphincter of Oddi.

Action   As with the treatment of the liver, the therapist also compresses the lower costal region from the lateral direction toward the patient's navel. With the other hand, the therapist attempts to contact the pyloric section of the stomach; the contact here is flat, avoiding the use of the fingertips. In a second treatment step, the therapist raises the pyloric section of the stomach as if in a small semicircle toward the lesser curvature of the stomach by moving both hands toward one another. In so doing, the therapist avoids the weight of the pyloric section affecting the upper section of the stomach and its ligamentous connection to the diaphragm. At this moment, the therapist somewhat reduces the compression on the ribcage and, by "listening," follows the upper section of the stomach to the end of its movement.

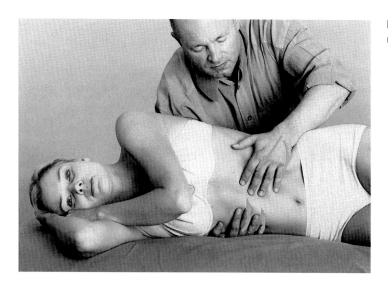

Figure 4.37 Treatment variation for the relationship between the liver and diaphragm.

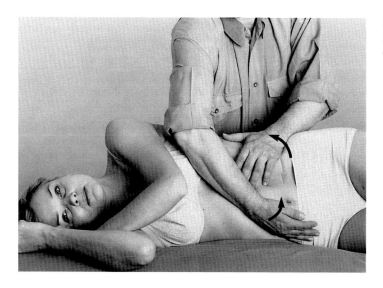

Figure 4.38 Treatment of the stomach in its relationship to the left cupula of the diaphragm.

Treatment of the relationship between the liver, stomach, diaphragm, and pleura

Patient Prone.

Therapist Standing to the side at the level of the hips.

Contact Precisely at the lower boundary of the ribs of the anterior chest cavity.

Action The therapist surrounds the lower thoracic cavity with both hands, avoiding placing strong pressure on any prominent or inelastic ribs. Both hands form precisely the arch of the individual ribs without exerting more pressure on one individual rib than on the others. The fingertips of both hands point in the direction of the xiphoid process. With both palms, the therapist now first compares the breathing motion on both sides. If a difference is discernible, the therapist uses the palm of the hand to try to sense the extent of the movement restriction. For this purpose, it is necessary to slightly modify the contact on both costal

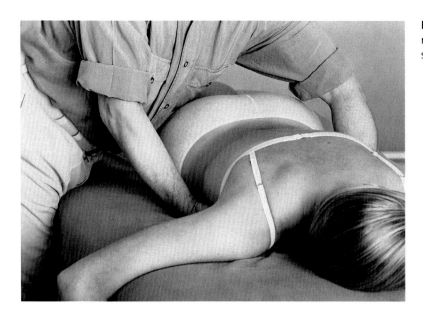

Figure 4.39 Treatment of the relationship between the liver, stomach, diaphragm, and pleura.

arches so as to ascertain whether the restriction of movement is located in the intercostal region, in the region of the organ connections toward the diaphragm, in the region of the connection between the diaphragm and the pleura located above it, or between the diaphragm and the pericardium. The therapist then compares the mobility of the various elements in relation to one another and tries to determine the spatial location of the most obvious restriction of movement. On the side of the most obvious restriction of movement, the therapist then gently compresses the ribcage toward the restriction of movement until a counterpressure is discernible. At this moment, the therapist reduces the pressure on the ribcage so that the countermotion can occur.

While the therapist increases the pressure on the chest cavity on the side of the restriction, the therapist also keeps the ribcage compressed on the other side with somewhat less exertion of pressure. This is necessary in order to prevent the fixation from escaping to the other side in the interior of the thorax. This technique also shows that it is possible to treat restrictions in the interior of a visceral cavity along with the adjacent myofascial exterior structure.

Treating the breathing pattern using globally applied spinal techniques

I have already referred several times to the fact that the sections of the body where the individual visceral cavities meet are of primary importance for the unrestricted motion of breathing. In the preceding chapters, techniques were described with which these regions can be treated from the front and lateral sides of the body. These techniques are intended to achieve an improved erect organization of the column of organs in the interior of the organism. However, they should also allow a more effortless alignment of the body along the line of gravity, so that less work must be done by the muscles to accomplish daily activities. In this sense, the techniques described above influence both the movement of the individual elements of the organism relative to one another and the structural constellations that result from this improved mobility at the same time. In the most favorable cases, they are simultaneously mobilizing and form-stabilizing techniques. As soon as we have achieved a more favorable alignment of the organ column, a response occurs in the region of the autonomic musculature of the back and ribcage.

The techniques described in this chapter concentrate on the fascial sheathing layers of the back musculature. They do not concentrate on the individual anatomical structures, however, but

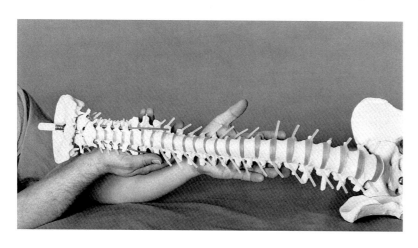

Figure 4.40 Hand position seen from the front.

attempt to influence the larger fascial network globally. For this purpose, it is technically necessary for us to evaluate the curves of the spine in its larger myofascial context. The following techniques can be described using a visual analogy similar to the one used in Chapter 1, which was a description of the technique used for the course of the nerves in the leg: we imagine the full, mobile interconnectedness of the vertebrae as a river, and all of the myofascial and ligamentous units surrounding this spine as the riverbed. The goal then is to influence the riverbed in such a way that a better flow pattern is achieved for the river.

It is crucial for the therapist's hands to be used in such a way that they touch the tissue structure at all of the contact points to the left and right of the spine. The goal is not to hold the spine in a fixed position because then correction with "listening" would not be possible. Rather, the goal is to relax the tissue bed of the spine by touching the major myofascial units in such a way that the tension pattern of the dominant minor myofascial and ligament units emerge more clearly.

Treatment of the curvature of the cervical and thoracic spine

Patient   Supine with legs extended.

Therapist   Sitting at the head.

Contact   With the palm of one hand on both sides of the spine at the level of the ninth thoracic vertebra, while the fingers of this hand, also on both sides of the spine, touch the tissue in the region below the ninth thoracic vertebra. The palm of the other hand very flexibly supports the occiput and the curve of the neck while the fingertips engage the tissue layer on both sides of the uppermost cervical vertebra.

Action   In the region of the thoracic spine, the therapist's hand adapts to the curve of the back. In so doing, the therapist takes care to emphasize the existing curvature of the thoracic spine. In the case of a severe kyphosis, the therapist follows the kyphosis in a somewhat more exaggerated curve. In the case of a pronounced flat back, the therapist follows into an even more exaggerated flat back. Subsequently, the therapist applies the same treatment strategy to the neck. In the case of a short, compressed neck with a strong lordotic curve, the therapist exaggerates this curve somewhat. In the case of a tendency toward hyperextension, the therapist's hands follow the hyperextension. Thus, the therapist reinforces the dominant curve pattern at both curvatures of the spine, in the region of the thoracic and cervical spine. It is now crucial for both curves to be amplified simultaneously. My assumption is that, in this way, we are able to induce a passive sliding of the dura within the spinal canal and perhaps even achieve a passive sliding of the perineurial sheaths.

Treatment of the transition between the thoracic spine and cervical spine and between the cervical spine and cranium

Patient   Supine, both legs flexed.

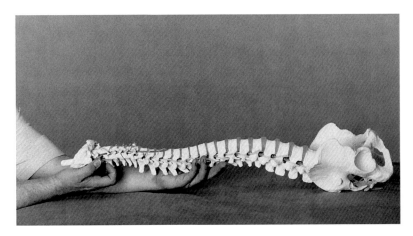

Figure 4.41 Lateral hand position.

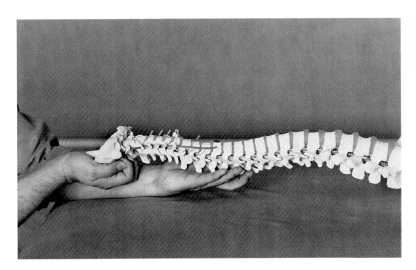

Figure 4.42 Treatment of the transition between the thoracic spine and cervical spine and between the cervical spine and cranium.

Therapist Sitting at the head.

Contact With the fingertips of one hand on both sides of the spine between the first and second ribs. The palm of the other hand supports the occiput and the fingers support the atlanto-occipital junction.

Action The therapist slightly raises the occiput until the dominant curvature of the cervical spine is more evident. In this technique as well, the dominant overall form of the neck is supported and very slightly exaggerated.

With the other hand, the therapist now precisely contacts the intermediate space between the first and second ribs using firm fingertip contact. This contact is made on both sides at the costovertebral connections. The therapist maintains this contact in a very flexible manner and prevents any sliding in the cranial direction. The patient rests on the therapist's fingertips as if bending backwards over the points of a garden fence. On the fascial level, this induces a stretching of the deep cervical fascia and, on the muscular level, an activation of the longus coli muscle. If this technique is correctly applied, the therapist can now detect how a shear effect at the transition point between the upper chest cavity and the anterior region of the neck is developing. The patient is given the impression that the neck is growing from the inside of the ribcage.

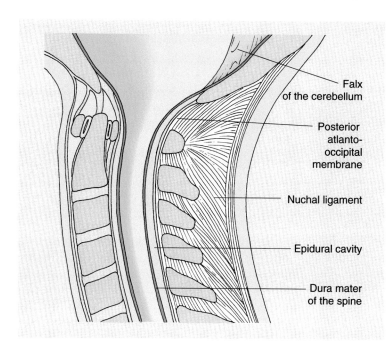

Figure 4.43   Fibrous path of the nuchal ligament.

Falx
of the cerebellum

Posterior
atlanto-
occipital
membrane

Nuchal ligament

Epidural cavity

Dura mater
of the spine

Most of the ligaments and muscular units in the region of the cervical spine have only a low level of intrinsic tension. For this reason, the entire cervical spine is significantly more mobile than the other sections of the spine. The technique described above does not access the small units, but rather the more extensive nuchal ligament. This band forms the bridge between the occiput and the upper back, where it joins with the fascia of the trapezius muscle. However, the nuchal ligament functions as a regulator of the mobility of the individual cervical vertebrae as well because it is directly connected to all of the spinous processes of the cervical spine. The tissue of this ligament has an extraordinarily high percentage of elastin. I assume that it is for this reason that it responds to subtle stretching.

Treatment of lumbar lordosis at the transition to the pelvic cavity

Patient   Supine with both legs extended.

Therapist   Standing at the level of the thigh.

Contact   In the case of a highly pronounced lordosis, one hand supports both sides of the lumbar spine. The other hand supports the sacrum. Even in the case of a straight lumbar spine with the typical curve between the last lumbar vertebra and the base of the sacrum, the therapist supports the sacrum with one hand, but the fingertips of the other hand reach on both sides of the spine into the narrow space between the transverse processes of the fourth lumbar vertebra, the sacrum, and both ilia.

Action   In the case of a hyperlordosis of the lumbar spine, the therapist intensifies the curve of the spine more and more from the posterior direction. At the same time, by supporting the sacrum, the therapist causes the pelvis to tilt more in the anterior direction along the axis of the hips. It is crucial that both hands be in strong contact with the tissue layers. This means that the hand at the level of the lumbar spine reaches strongly into the tissue next to the transverse processes and intensifies the curve of the spine until a countermovement is felt. Then the therapist does not yet allow the lumbar spine to return from the exaggerated lordosis, but rather first allows the sacrum or the entire section of the pelvis to sink back somewhat from the exaggerated anterior tilt, while an strong pull is exerted on the lumbar fascia. The therapist subsequently allows

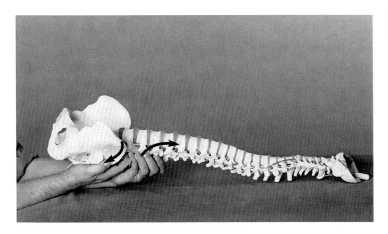

Figure 4.44 Treatment of lumbar lordosis at the transition to the pelvic cavity.

the middle of the lumbar spine to slowly return to the posterior position, i.e. the exaggerated lordotic curve is reduced farther. The therapist remains in contact with the layers of tissue running next to the lumbar spine in such a way that a pull or, even better, a shear effect is exerted in the cranial direction.

This technique for treating hyperlordosis of the lumbar spine may be divided into two steps. In one step, the therapist intensifies the curve of the lumbar spine and the anterior tilt of the pelvis on the hip axis. In a second step, the therapist guides the patient's back and pelvis out of the exaggerated lordosis and out of the exaggerated pelvic tilt back into their usual position and then beyond it. It is crucial that, at the moment in which the spine reduces its usual lordotic bend, a strong stretching of the lower portion of the lumbar fascia is achieved in the distal direction. Using the fingertips, it should be stretched in such a way that only a minimal sliding motion of a few millimeters occurs between the therapist's hand and the surface of the fascia. At the same time, the hand applied to the lumbar spine produces a subtle stretching of the thoracolumbar fascia in the opposite, i.e. cranial, direction.

Treatment of flat back of the lumbar spine

In the case of flat back in the lumbar region, hardly any curve is visible at all. However, we usually find a kink on the radiograph between the lumbar spine, which is running straight without a curve, and the sacrum, which is located between the two alae of the ilium. The following technique intensifies the kink between the sacrum and the fifth lumbar vertebra in order to then reduce it gradually such that the hypertonically pronounced tension pattern of this very small area is distributed over larger sections of the lumbar spine.

Patient Supine, both legs extended.

Therapist Standing at the level of the thigh.

Contact With flat contact on the sacrum with one hand, contact with single spots in the region between the fourth and fifth lumbar vertebra and the upper boundary of the pelvis using the tips of the fingers and thumb of the other hand.

Action This time, the therapist provides only a gentle impulse in the direction of the stronger anterior tilting of the sacrum, while the other hand reaches in the anterior direction on both sides through the muscle layers near the spine in the direction of the iliolumbar ligaments. In a second treatment step, the therapist then minimally alters the tilt of the pelvis on the hip axis several times using the hand supporting the sacrum, while maintaining the contact with the other hand in the direction of the iliolumbar ligaments, i.e. in the direction of the connection between the fourth lumbar vertebra and both alae of the ilium. If this technique is performed correctly, the fifth lumbar vertebra now comes to be suspended between the two hands of the therapist. The therapist tries to exploit this state of suspension by allowing a sort

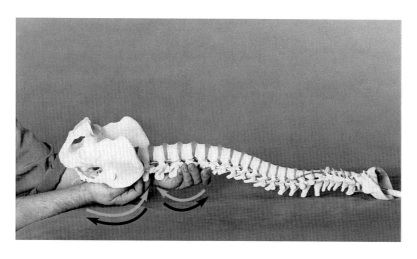

Figure 4.45 Treatment of flat back of the lumbar spine.

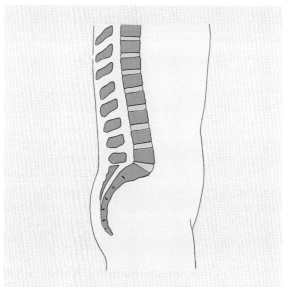

Figure 4.46 Flat back of the lumbar spine.

of passive traction between the fifth lumbar vertebra and the sacrum, i.e. precisely in the kink. The therapist gradually attempts to transmit the forces of this passive traction into the large superficial layers along the entire lumbar spine.

Treatment of posterior tilting of the pelvis using the myofascial tension paths on the rear of the thigh

The manner in which the pelvis tilts in the anterior or posterior direction on the hip axis depends greatly on how the myofascial layers of the lower

extremities act on the inferior aspects of the pelvis. At the ischial tuberosity, the tensile forces of the biceps femoris muscle unite with the tough layers of the sacrotuberous ligament. The resulting myofascial–ligamentous unit is an essential factor in the tilting of the pelvis in the posterior direction on the hip axis. Increased tension in the ligaments mentioned above prevents the natural yielding of both tuberosities when sitting and supports the tendency of both ilia to open in an "out-flare." This is a movement of the ilium in the frontal plane in which the iliac crest wanders in the lateral direction and the ischial tuberosity in the medial direction. At the same time, myofascial tension patterns of the biceps femoris do not allow the tuberosities to slide far enough in the posterior direction when sitting. Because the myofascial units mentioned above and the band structure form an inseparable tension unit, this leads to a narrowing of the lower pelvic cavity. We can only speculate whether this reduction of space has a negative effect on the exchange of fluids or metabolic processes of the organs located in this region. I particularly expect a negative effect for the prostate and how it moves in relation to the bladder.

Any treatment of a posterior pelvic tilt should begin with a treatment of the tension patterns of the lower extremity (cf. the technique for the treatment of the fascia lata found in the section on the lower extremity and, in particular, the techniques for treatment of the fasciae of the adductor group, see section 4.5). This technique builds on the extremity techniques mentioned above and attempts to

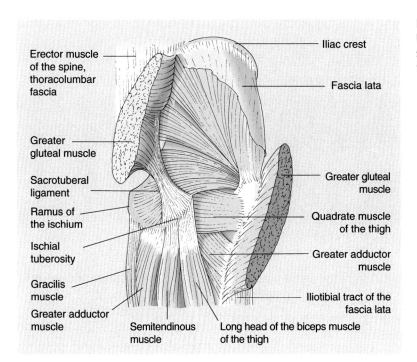

Erector muscle of the spine, thoracolumbar fascia

Greater gluteal muscle

Sacrotuberal ligament

Ramus of the ischium

Ischial tuberosity

Gracilis muscle

Greater adductor muscle

Semitendinous muscle

Long head of the biceps muscle of the thigh

Iliac crest

Fascia lata

Greater gluteal muscle

Quadrate muscle of the thigh

Greater adductor muscle

Iliotibial tract of the fascia lata

Figure 4.47   Connection between the biceps femoris muscle and the sacrotuberous ligament at the ischial tuberosity.

make their effect in the region of the lumbosacral transition more precise.

Patient   Lying on one side.

Therapist   Standing at the level of the hips.

Contact   With the fingertips of one hand just below the ischial tuberosity, precisely between the origins of the biceps femoris muscle and the semi-tendinosus muscle, and with the outside edge of the other hand gently contacting the superior edge of the ala of the ilium in the direction of the ilio-lumbar ligament.

Action   The therapist first reaches between the biceps femoris and the semimembranosus muscle slightly below its origin and attempts to arrive between the fascial sheaths of both muscular units. It is not easy to differentiate both of these muscular units in this area since it contains multiple tendon origins. However, it is necessary to reach precisely in the intermediate space between both fascial sheaths because experience shows that contact which provides direction is sufficient to produce a response from the tissue. With the other hand, the therapist moves the upper portion of the ilium

slightly farther into the out-flare. Experience shows that the tuberosity on the lower edge of the pelvis moves somewhat toward the contralateral tuberosity. Both of the therapist's hands follow the movement of the ala of the ilium, while the contact between the biceps femoris and the semitendi-nosus muscle continues unabated. As soon as the movement into the out-flare has reached its end-point, the therapist considerably intensifies the contact between the two muscles below the ischial tuberosity until a new direction of motion is sensed: the therapist accompanies the upper edge of the pelvis in the direction of an in-flare and, at the same time, moves the tuberosity in a very slight spreading motion. In the in-flare, the ilium moves in the frontal plane and the iliac crest wanders in the medial direction and the ischial tuberosity in the lateral direction.

Combined treatment of posterior pelvic tilt and out-flare of the ilium on both sides

Patient   Prone, ankles extending over the lower edge of the treatment table.

Therapist   Standing at the level of the thigh.

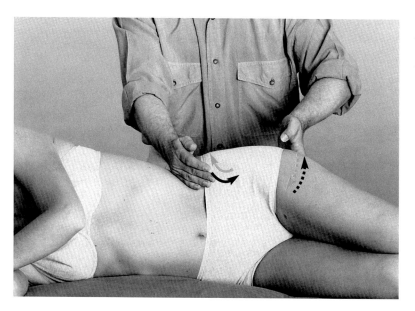

Figure 4.48   Treatment of posterior tilting of the pelvis using the myofascial tension paths behind the thigh.

Contact   With the erect foremost fingertips of both hands beneath the fourth segment of the sacrum.

Action   The therapist ensures that the patient's legs are parallel to one another and are not rotated outward. The therapist then makes contact at the level of the fourth segment of the sacrum bilaterally from the center line of the sacrum. In so doing, it is essential for the touch to press persistently through the subcutaneous fatty layer in order to reach the interosseus sacroiliac ligaments located on both sides at this point. This band structure is located under the dense fiber network of the lumbar fascia adhering to the sacrum. The contact should be as if trying to release the lumbar fascia from its connection with the ligament's structure beneath it. In a second treatment step, the therapist then begins to exert pressure in the cranial direction with the fingertips of both hands while avoiding pushing the sacrum anteriorly. The therapist matches the arch of the bone precisely, but remains in extremely intense contact with the lower fascial layers surrounding the sacrum from the posterior direction and embedding it in the overall formation of the back. The quality of the contact should be gradually intensified as if the periosteum, i.e. the layer located below the interosseus sacroiliac ligament, were being pushed onto the bone in the cranial direction. Experience shows us that the patient will experience a mild,

burning pain. This extremely intense action should be made up to slightly below the upper edge of the sacrum while, as mentioned above, preventing the base of the sacrum from tilting forward. While pushing in a cranial direction, the therapist modifies the very slow speed of movement so that it is possible, through "listening," to detect how both ilia are released somewhat from the constant tension of the interosseus sacroiliac ligaments and are wandering from their fixed out-flare position in the direction of an in-flare.

When the therapist applies the contact with a very flat angle, i.e. almost parallel to the arch of the sacrum, a pulling effect occurs on the posterior side of the tailbone in the inferior direction, which continues to the superficial posterior sacrococcygeal ligament. If the therapist follows this pull effect deeper with "listening," it is possible to influence the tension patterns in their connection to the dura mater. In the case of a very lasting effect on the ligament's connections between the sacrum and both ilia, the technique described above is also suitable for correction of strongly pronounced knock knee.

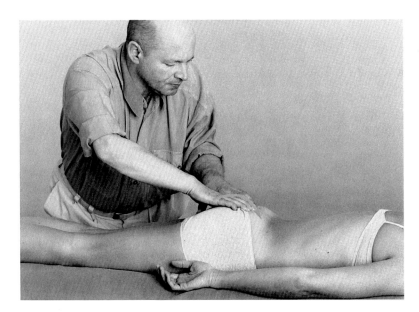

Figure 4.49 Combined treatment of posterior pelvic tilt and out-flare of the ilium on both sides.

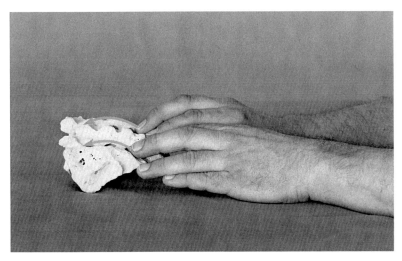

Figure 4.50 Positions of the fingers on the sacrum.

Treatment of flat back in the thoracic spine

Patient Supine, legs extended.

Therapist Sitting at the head.

Contact With one hand on both sides of the spine at the level of the sixth thoracic vertebra, while the other palm supports the occiput and the fingers produce contact at the transition between the atlas and occipital bone.

Action It is a precondition for the efficacy of this technique that the therapist be able to place one supporting hand under the back in such a way that

the habitual flat back of the thoracic spine is not altered. The contact must be kept flat with the palm of the hand; in other words, the patient's spine is resting in the hand of the therapist, who produces additional contact with the layers of tissue near the spine using the fingertips. The therapist uses the other hand to hold the occiput in such a way that the spatial relationship between the head, neck, and chest cavity approximates the spatial relationship displayed by the patient when standing. The therapist then allows the patient's head to sink minimally in the posterior direction, i.e. toward the treatment table, but avoids any pull on the cervical

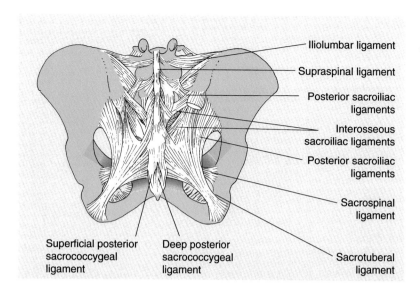

Figure 4.51   Pelvic bone and its ligamentous connections in the female from the posterior.

Iliolumbar ligament

Supraspinal ligament

Posterior sacroiliac ligaments

Interosseous sacroiliac ligaments

Posterior sacroiliac ligaments

Sacrospinal ligament

Sacrotuberal ligament

Superficial posterior sacrococcygeal ligament

Deep posterior sacrococcygeal ligament

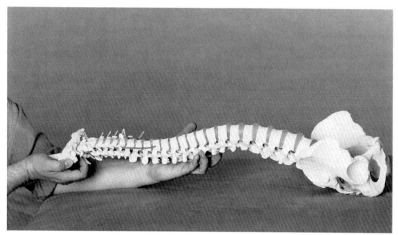

Figure 4.52   Treatment of flat back in the thoracic spine.

spine. Under no circumstances should strong traction forces be acting on the neck. At the same time, the therapist's other palm supports the spine in the thoracic region somewhat more, such that the flat back in this region becomes more pronounced. In addition, the therapist places the fingertips strongly into the tissue to the left and right of the thoracic spine. As soon as the therapist is able to feel the thoracic spine trying to move even a little bit out of the flat back in the direction of a natural kyphotic bend, the therapist follows and intensifies this movement. In so doing, it is important that the therapist respond to and emphasize the three-dimensional structure of this movement of the vertebral bodies, i.e. rotations and side tilts, even in their smallest

manifestations. Before and after the application of this technique, it is worth examining the affected section of the spine with joint tests to verify the efficacy of this technique (Barral *et al.* 1993).

Treatment of exaggerated kyphosis of the thoracic spine

Patient   Lying on one side with flexed knees.

Therapist   Standing at the level of the hips.

Contact   Depending on the tone of the tissue, with the flat front phalanges of both hands, gently used edges of the hand, or the palms.

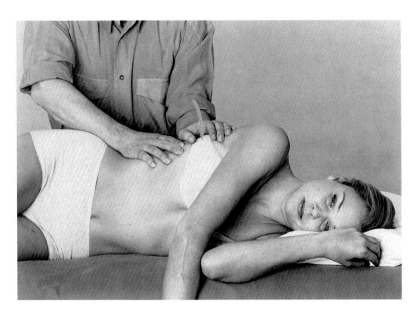

Figure 4.53   Treatment of exaggerated kyphosis of the thoracic spine.

Action   In order to guarantee the efficacy of this technique, we must rely on the patient's active participation. While the therapist makes contact in the lateral portion of the ribcage approximately at the level of the sixth rib, the patient allows the arm on this side to hang over the edge of the treatment table. The therapist examines the density of the various fascial layers in this region. It is possible that the therapist will find a large density of fibers on the surface, possibly at the lateral boundary of the fascia of the latissimus dorsi muscle and its connection to the upper arm, or possibly not until the fascial connective layer between the serratus anterior and the oblique abdominal muscle, or in the intercostal region. The therapist uses both hands and intensifies the contact simultaneously posterior and anterior of the lateral midline of the torso. It is important to ensure that the shear effect in the cranial direction acts on the surface only to the extent that the layers located below can follow the stretching effect. The goal is not a mechanically local effect on the side of the ribcage, but rather more of a solution for the three-dimensional connection between the shoulder and chest cavity. For this reason, it is necessary for the patient's arm to be allowed to hang from the treatment table with more and more weight during manual treatment as if the patient were reaching for an object on the floor.

Coordinated treatment of strongly pronounced kyphosis of the thoracic spine

Patient   Sitting on a bench with thighs parallel to one another.

Therapist   Standing to the side next to the patient.

Contact   Supporting the sternum with one palm from the anterior direction, at the same time making contact with the other hand on both sides of the thoracic spine, approximately at the level of the sixth thoracic vertebra

Action   The therapist asks the patient to maintain good contact between the feet and the floor. While supporting the chest cavity from the anterior and posterior sides, the therapist applies a very gentle impulse in the cranial direction, as if to lift the ribcage away from the abdominal and pelvic cavities. At the same time, the therapist asks the patient to completely relax the abdominal wall so that the pelvis is tilting slightly forward. Subsequently, the patient should intensify contact with the floor somewhat so that the pelvis sinks back into its starting position and slightly into the posterior position. This sequence of movements should be repeated several times. The therapist registers the shear effect in the region of the chest cavity caused by the motion of the pelvis, and influences the tissue

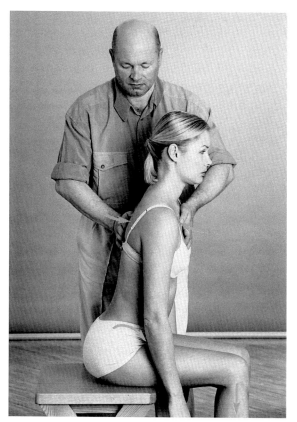

Figure 4.54 Coordinated treatment of strongly pronounced kyphosis of the thoracic spine.

the region of the third thoracic vertebra, avoiding a pull effect in the cranial direction. The therapist structures the quality of the touch so that the patient receives the impression of being subtly flexed backward at the level of the third thoracic vertebra. At the same moment, the therapist exaggerates the hyperextension of the cervical spine to a minimal extent and the therapist's entire attention is directed toward the instant when the entire neck tries to move out of the hyperextension into a slight bend. The therapist supports this movement with subtle contact with both hands, visualizing the connection of the nuchal ligament to the occiput and of the individual spinous processes of the cervical spine in the connection of the nuchal ligament to the fascia of the trapezius muscle.

> Under all circumstances, the therapist must prevent the dragging forces from acting on the neck since raw muscular force will mask the fine pull effect of the highly elastic nuchal ligament. Visually, the therapist treats the nuchal ligament like a flat cord to which the spine and spinous processes are connected. The therapist's attention is directed at two levels of "listening": on the one hand, at the overall tension pattern between the upper chest cavity, neck, and base of the skull and, on the other hand, at the joint connections, i.e. the detailed structure of the neck.

from the posterior direction precisely below the most discernible bilateral facet fixations.

Treatment of a chronically hyperextended neck

Patient Supine with both legs extended.

Therapist Sitting at the head.

Contact With the fingers of one hand on both sides of the upper thoracic spine, at the level of the third thoracic vertebra, while the second hand supports the occiput.

Action The therapist first raises the occiput a small distance from the treatment table, but only far enough to maintain the present hyperextension of the cervical spine. Then the therapist initiates contact with the tissue on both sides of the spine in

Treatment of chronically contracted myofascial layers of the neck

Patient Supine with both legs flexed.

Therapist Standing at the head, one flexed knee resting on the lowered treatment table.

Contact While one hand raises the occiput, the other hand initiates a flat contact with the layers posterior to the sternocleidomastoid muscle. The therapist's elbow rests on the flexed knee in order to keep the patient's head at a relatively high level.

Action It is important for the patient's neck to be slightly rotated and flexed to the side to be treated, so that the exterior layers are sufficiently relaxed.

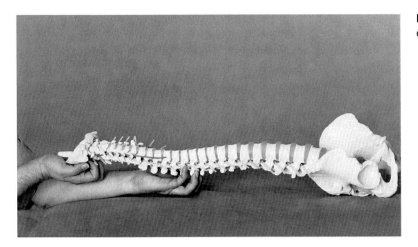

Figure 4.55 Treatment of a chronically hyperextended neck.

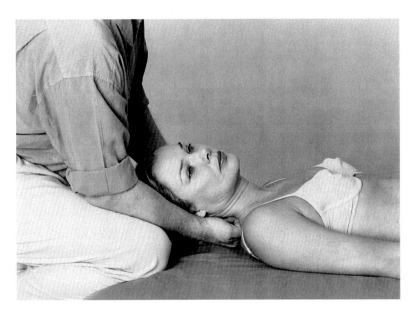

Figure 4.56 Treatment of chronically contracted myofascial layers of the neck.

Here, it is crucial for the therapist to be able to penetrate between the trapezius muscle and sternocleidomastoid muscle to the middle scalene muscle. As soon as the middle scalene muscle is contacted, the therapist intensifies the quality of the touch and begins to slide the hand in the direction of the muscle origin to the side of the cervical spine. Thus, the therapist's hand is moving diagonally, i.e. in the mediocranial direction. By slightly changing the position of the head by increasing or decreasing the neck's rotation and/or curve to the side, layers at different depths may be accessed. This technique should be applied to both sides; it is important to keep in mind that the intensity of the touch is modified relative to the tension that is present.

This technique may be varied in relation to the shape of the neck. If the neck appears contracted in all of its levels, i.e. in the superficial fascia, deep fascia, and myofascial layers, it is advisable to create contact with the scalene muscle selectively rather than with the flat hand. This works especially well in male patients with highly pronounced muscle tone, with the therapist bending the index and middle fingers of one hand and acting very specifically on the scalene fascia. It is important to avoid placing pressure on the vessels. The portion of the brachial plexus running under the clavicle should be treated carefully here as well and under no circumstances should it be pressed against the transverse processes of the cervical spine. As long as only a short-term, careful stretching effect is directed at the connective tissue coat of the plexus, a positive effect will result because the nerve has thus found its natural basic tension in relationship to its boundary layers.

4.2   MYOFASCIAL TREATMENT OF SCOLIOSIS

In orthopedics, the appearance of scoliosis is primarily examined using radiological imaging. The diagnosis and prognosis are concentrated on the registration of the angle of curvature of individual sections of the spine. To a certain extent, this diagnostic procedure provides information about the deviation from the norm that is present in the curve of the spine. However, the measuring procedure used in these cases is not very reliable because radiology is only capable of showing a three-dimensional curve in two dimensions. In addition, radiological imaging provides only a momentary picture that does not allow a reading of fluctuations in the relevant curvature that may be caused by breathing and changes in posture. For this reason, I doubt that a long-term prognosis regarding the stability of the back or the guarantee of respiratory volume and the space for functional cardiac activity can be made using the traditional imaging procedure.

From the perspective of the myofascial concept, scoliosis appears not only as an irregular curvature of the spine that manifests in three dimensions, but also as an altered spatial relationship of the visceral cavities and a very stable spatial displacement of individual organ axes. This perspective can be supported by the fact that, from a manual diagnostic standpoint, the tendencies to develop scoliosis may be diagnosed in the early years of life before the scoliotic curve manifests in the spine. Manual diagnosis provides insight into altered tension relationships of the membranes that cover the visceral cavities. These altered tension relationships may be found within the craniosacral membrane system as well as in the connective tissue groups of the abdominal and pelvic cavities.

In the past two decades, I have had repeated opportunities to observe the long-term development of scoliosis in cooperation with pediatricians and orthopedists, beginning with infancy. Our observations do not claim the validity of a scientific study, but they do suggest a reevaluation of the traditional view of scoliosis, which is focused on the diagnosis of the spine and back.

The observations we were able to make of so-called idiopathic scoliosis in infancy were particularly illuminating. The children were brought to us because their mothers had pronounced scoliosis; in some cases, scoliosis was present in three generations. Even though no irregular curvatures of the spine were observed in orthopedic examinations of the infants, we were able to discover altered pull forces of the dura mater on the cranium and the sacrum in our manual examinations. In a manner of speaking, we found scoliotic tendencies anchored in the deep membranes as early as the first weeks of life. Our diagnosis was confirmed in subsequent years: all of the children we had diagnosed ultimately developed spinal curvatures that could be diagnosed by radiography.

Based on our observations, we drew the conclusion that scoliotic patterns can be manifest at a point in time when the tonal forces of the musculature are weakly developed, i.e. substantially earlier than at ten or eleven years old, when it becomes particularly obvious due to the child's increased growth in height. Thus, at least in some cases, scoliosis cannot be attributed to irregular muscle forces in the back. Rather, it could be considered a result of an unusual growth behavior of the myofascial system which causes disorientation of muscle tone as a secondary effect. This assumption can be supported by the fact that it is the connective tissue and not the central nervous system that primarily supports the growth processes of the organism.

It is not simple to make general statements on the etiology of scoliosis solely on the basis of individual cases. However, our diagnostic observations, along with the practical results of the treatment techniques we used, at least provide a starting point when reconsidering the traditional diagnosis and treatment of scoliosis.

We must observe that the form of the spine diagnosed as scoliosis obviously arises from fundamentally different causes. In many cases, a genetic disposition is obviously present. In other cases, however, these genetic factors do not have a role and in other cases it was an unusual position of the fetus during development which apparently caused a change in the membrane structure in the interior of the visceral cavities, especially in the area of the chest cavity and within the craniosacral system. Finally, we encounter the cases that are relevant to the treatment technique we describe, namely the cases that display a drastic displacement of the axes of mobility of the organs located below the diaphragm.

In most of such cases that we have investigated, the stomach plays an important role. In the section that examined the significance of the breathing pattern (section 4.1), we have seen that the dynamics of the breathing process will fashion and stabilize the chest cavity. All pronounced changes in the mobility of an organ on one side of the diaphragm will influence the chest cavity. As we can see, this sort of altered spatial excursion of the diaphragm and lung occurs on the same side. Here, altered rotational forces are acting from the anterior direction on entire groups of thoracic vertebrae; as soon as one cupula of the diaphragm has the tendency to be in permanent descent, the joints within the back must compensate for this descent with a corresponding lateral bend. To a lesser extent, similar influences are conceivable if an infection within the chest cavity has caused one-sided adhesions on the connective layers of the thoracic wall. A displacement of the axis in the lung area occurs that follows the reshaped thoracic wall. In this manner, the shape of both halves of the chest can change drastically.

However, in relation to this, the subdiaphragmatic organs appear to be of greater significance in influencing the curvatures of the spine. So it is important to examine both cupulas of the diaphragm carefully for their spatial relationships

and mobility relative to the organs. In so doing, we should focus our attention on the elastic capacity of the intercostal membranes and the subcostal myofascial layers as well.

During embryonic development, all of the organs undergo a characteristic shift in position, a type of "voyage through space," until they arrive at their destination within the interior of the visceral cavities. In practice, we can see that there is at least one common type of scoliosis that can be attributed to an incomplete spatial curve of the stomach. In this case, the back appears to be sunken in the upper left lumbar region and the vertebrae above it display the typical scoliotic curvature such that the entire upper body appears to have been displaced to the right in relation to the pelvis.

At first glance, there appears to be an imbalance in tone of the erector muscles, and the latissimus dorsi muscle is indeed usually very weakly developed on the left side. The muscular support of the quadratus lumborum muscle that spans the upper crest of the pelvis and the lower edge of the twelfth rib appears hardly present at all.

If we direct our attention to the examination of the prevertebral region, we also find a drastically altered spatial position of the stomach in relation to the midline of the body. Apparently, in these cases, the stomach did not completely follow the spatial curve intended for it during embryonic development. For this reason, it is located more medially compared with its normal position and therefore can provide only minimal support for the left cupula of the diaphragm. Its relationship to the spleen is altered in the cranial direction and its relationship to the left kidney in the inferior direction. Therefore, on the right side of the thorax, a stable support is present from the liver, which is "denser" than the stomach. The left cupula of the diaphragm drops and, as I assume, the formation of the typical scoliotic curvature occurs in the sections of the spine located over it.

Unfortunately, in this sort of situation, I was able to achieve very few results with treatment techniques applied to the back. There is even the danger that manual influence on the myofascial layers of the scoliotically curved back could cause a destabilization of individual joint sections. In contrast, a subdiaphragmatic, i.e. visceral, procedure is consistently able to provide satisfactory results, in particular when we select the treatment strategy that accompanies the child's growth process over a longer period of time with minimal interventions.

Treatment of scoliosis in infancy and until the third year of life

Small child   Resting with the occiput on one of the therapist's hands and the pelvis on the other hand.

Therapist   Standing, one leg flexed on a footstool or the lowered treatment table.

Contact   The therapist's forearm is supported on the flexed knee while holding the child's pelvis so that the legs fall to the side next to the therapist's forearm. At the same time, the therapist supports the occiput.

Action   The therapist follows bimanually on the pelvis and cranium while "listening," initially without exerting a pull on the dura. If a tendency toward scoliosis is present, both of the therapist's hands, at the pelvis and cranium, will twist slightly relative to one another. It is now essential to first intensify this twisting tendency while exerting traction on the dura and the adjacent layers and to follow the motion until it comes to rest. The traction should first be intensified and then slowly reduced in such a way that the pelvis and occiput move back out of their twisted position. This entire sequence of movements should be repeated three or four times; it is important to ensure that the traction exerted by the therapist's hands acts on the layers near the spine and the layers of the interior spinal canal, avoiding a stretching of the superficial layers.

The efficacy of the technique described above increases if we first perform a preliminary treatment on the child using craniosacral techniques on the transition between the upper cervical spine and the base of the skull and at the transition between the lumbar spine and sacrum. This guarantees that the growth in length at both ends of the spine can occur, minimizing the myofascial and ligamentous blockages in this region (see the depiction in Upledger and Vredevoogd 1983: 268–9).

Treatment of scoliosis in adults

Patient   Sitting on a stool.

Therapist   Standing behind the patient with the right knee flexed on the stool while the patient's

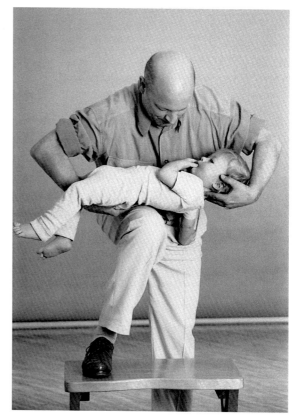

Figure 4.57   Treatment of scoliosis in infancy and until the third year of life.

upper arm is placed on the therapist's knee and is supported that way.

Contact   With the left hand on the stomach and the right hand on the costal arch.

Action   The therapist guides the patient's upper body into a somewhat more pronounced curve. At the same time, the therapist's left hand surrounds the stomach from below and raises it in the cranial direction, precisely in the direction of its band attachment near the center line of the body. In so doing, the therapist surrounds the left costal arch so that the fingers maintain contact with the stomach while the palm compresses the ribcage in a diagonal direction toward the xiphoid process. A slight increase occurs in the existing scoliotic curve; the right half of the thorax rotates in the anterior direction around the central axis of the right lung. At this moment, the therapist's right hand compresses the right half of the thorax as well at the level of the sixth rib so that the pressure is transmitted in the cranial direction. This movement should occur so that the stomach continues to be lifted in the direction of its band fixation, the right half of the thorax is being compressed from the front like a drum during rotation, and the thorax as a whole is moved in the cranial direction as if it were being lifted off of the pelvic cavity. Subsequently, the therapist allows the patient's upper body to sink toward the pelvis again and guides it back into the normal position.

> The technique is applied simultaneously to the left subdiaphragmal space and the inner layers of the right half of the thorax at the level of the sixth rib. Thus, it affects the support of the left cupula of the diaphragm by the stomach on one side. The technique also has influence on the connecting layer between the serratus anterior muscle and the oblique abdominal muscle at the exterior of the ribcage, the intercostal membranes and myofascial subcostal layers and the parietal pleura in the interior. Here, it is crucial that the direct pressure on myofascial layers be applied to the exterior structure of the ribcage with precise indirect treatment between the organ and diaphragm simultaneously. With this technique as well, it is advisable to perform prior treatments on the atlanto-occipital transition (see section 5.1) and the transition between the lumbar spine and the sacrum (see section 5.1) and to perform the same treatments again after the technique described above.

If the scoliotic curvature of the thoracic spine is primarily manifest in the left thoracic cavity, it is possible to modify the technique described for the relationship between the stomach and diaphragm (see section 4.1) correspondingly for the transition from the liver to the right cupula of the diaphragm.

The goal of the scoliosis treatment described here is not to straighten the spine, but rather to improve mobility in the deep membranes in which the curvatures of the spine are embedded. Naturally, if the techniques described above are applied correctly, the extreme scoliotic curvature will be reduced. However, it is essential that the back develop

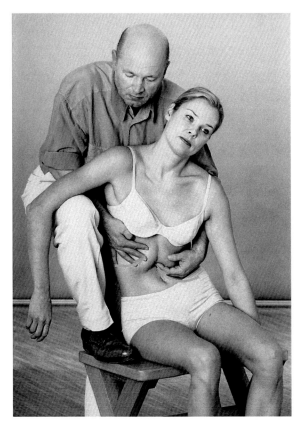

Figure 4.58   Treatment of scoliosis in adults.

toward symmetry only as far as it is reflected by the position and mobility of the organs. In my opinion, any treatment on one side applied only to the back will only intensify the discrepancy between the pre- and postvertebral components of the back.

4.3   THE SHOULDER GIRDLE: THE BRIDGE TO THE UPPER EXTREMITY

Aspects of form

In anatomical literature, the shoulder joint is described as the most mobile joint of the human body. Thanks to its mobility, it is easily able to compensate for shear and pull forces that are statically caused and originate from other sections of the upper body. These forces arise from normal differences between each side of the thorax, and these differences arise from an asymmetrical interior structure of the thoracic cavity. They do not necessarily cause functional disruptions unless the exceed a critical threshold.

There are a great many differences between sides that act on the pectoral girdle. Their roots may be traced into the pelvis and down into the lower extremities. However, we are most frequently confronted by differences in respiratory dynamics. In such cases, the basis for the difference between sides lies either in the interior of the ribcage or in the region of the transition between the abdominal cavity and chest cavity. If the movement patterns of breathing are restricted on one side near the diaphragm, the dynamic foundation of one half of the thorax is altered (see section 4.1). In order to maintain equilibrium in gravity, the tonus pattern of the muscles will compensate around a shoulder joint. As a long-term process, this change will ultimately lead to changes in the affected fascial layers. Low-fluid, fibrous components of connective tissue will predominate when compared with the layers containing elastin. If this process continues, a conflict arises between mobility and stability of the shoulder joint. The joint builds the bridge between a huge range of vectors of motion of the arm and the relatively static process of ensuring respiratory volume in the upper chest cavity. In order to guarantee respiratory volume, the fascial system needs, on the one hand, tough anchors that surround the joint as a whole and anchor it in the posterior direction; on the other hand, sliding layers must be present to allow the spatial displacements of the scapula that are necessary in order to move the arms.

The use of our arms occurs mostly in the front and lateral regions; only rarely do we reach behind ourselves. In quadrupeds, the upper respiratory space is automatically guaranteed because it virtually hangs from the dorsal portion of the pectoral girdle. When an organism is standing upright, this automatic maintenance of respiratory space is lost. Under the influence of gravity, the pectoral girdle compresses the upper respiratory space. Both functions of the shoulders—securing a stable respiratory space and allowing a large radius of movement for the arm—can be fulfilled only if an equilibrium is present between the tough and the sliding fascial layers. In order to locate the seams of this equilibrium, it is necessary to take a look at the fascial structure of the shoulders.

Anatomy of the fasciae

If we consider the anterior connections between the ribcage, pectoral girdle, and upper arm, the dominance of the pectoralis major is striking. This muscle has a multitude of tasks to fulfill: it is involved in all inner rotations and adductions of the arm and it is responsible for a considerable portion of force transmission in raising the arm. Moreover, with fibers running in three different directions, it can raise the pectoral girdle, lower it, and move it in the medial direction.

Its fascia, the pectoral fascia, is anchored at bone and connective tissue connections. It is connected to the clavicle in the cranial direction, to the sternum in the medial direction, and to the fascia of the ala in the dorsal direction. In comparison with the muscle, which is often quite hefty, especially in men, the fascia is relatively thin, has a rather fine tissue character, and is easily moved, both outward toward the skin as well as toward the deep layer located under it.

In contrast to the fascia of the pectoralis major, the fascia of the pectoralis minor is usually much stronger and tougher. The difference in the structure of the two fasciae plays an essential role in the treatment of the shoulder joint: it is not the fascia of the large chest muscle that is a deciding factor in restricting movement of the shoulder joint, but rather the fascia of the smaller muscle. The reason for this is that the clavipectoral fascia surrounds the pectoralis minor as well as the subclavius and the coracobrachialis muscles. In other words, the clavipectoral fascia simultaneously regulates the radius of action of the muscular connections between the pectoral girdle and the ribcage as well as between the pectoral girdle and the arm.

In the deeper layers, the fascia of the pectoralis minor is connected with the capsule of the shoulder joint. Moreover, it is in contact with the envelope of the brachial plexus. Thus, along with some fibers, this fascia is responsible for the connection of the ribcage to the interior structure of the shoulder joint, while guaranteeing segmented connection between the ribcage and pectoral girdle along with other fibers. In conjunction with the fascia of the subclavius and the coracobrachialis muscles, the fascia of the pectoralis minor fulfills the following function as the clavipectoral fascia: it acts as a fascial bridge

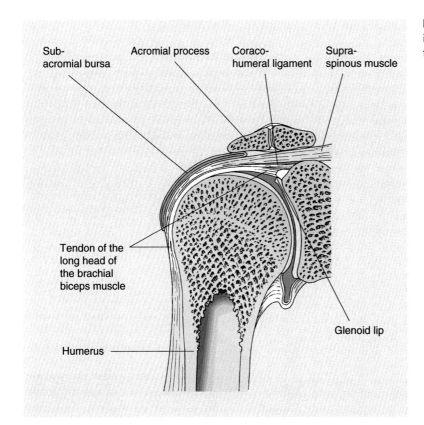

Sub-acromial bursa

Acromial process

Coraco-humeral ligament

Supra-spinous muscle

Tendon of the long head of the brachial biceps muscle

Glenoid lip

Humerus

Figure 4.59 *Supraspinatus muscle in interaction with the biceps muscle of the arm.*

between the pectoral girdle and the ribcage, running between the third, fourth, and fifth ribs to the coracoid process of the scapula (route of the pectoralis minor) and from the first rib to the clavicle (route of the subclavius muscle), as well as the fascial bridge that runs between the shoulder and upper arm from the coracoid process and to the crest of the lesser tubercule (route of the coracobrachialis muscle).

If we now turn our attention to behind the pectoral girdle, we also find a particularly strongly pronounced fascia that forms the counterpoint to the clavipectoral fascia: the fascia infraspinata. It is attached to the spine and at the lateral margin of the scapula and surrounds the infraspinatus muscle with its various fibrous directions along with the teres minor muscle. The fascia infraspinata not only serves as a muscular sheath, but also functions as an attachment for the muscle fibers in places, in particular in the region of the vertebral border of the scapula.

Furthermore, similar conditions are also present in the supraspinatus muscle above the infraspinatus

muscle. As a muscle, the supraspinatus has a less sturdy structure than the infraspinatus, in contrast to their fasciae. Spanning the capsule of the shoulder joint, the supraspinatus muscle has an important function. For this reason, its fascia also plays an essential role in our treatment technique.

In practice, it is important to keep in mind that only the teres minor muscle lies inside the fascia infraspinata. The teres major muscle is outside it, in a common fascial sheath with the latissimus dorsi muscle.

If we now include the costal side of the scapula in our consideration, we encounter the fascial sheath of the subscapularis muscle. Its fascial sheath also has a sturdy structure and, in addition, is loosely displaceable. By means of this layer, it is possible for the scapula to make sliding movements on the torso.

In the literature, the cooperation of the scapulohumeral fasciae as a flat configuration of connective tissue is described. This disk of connective tissue is important because it surrounds the entire muscular

Figure 4.60 Path of the subdeltoid fascia (horizontal cross-section of the shoulder joint).

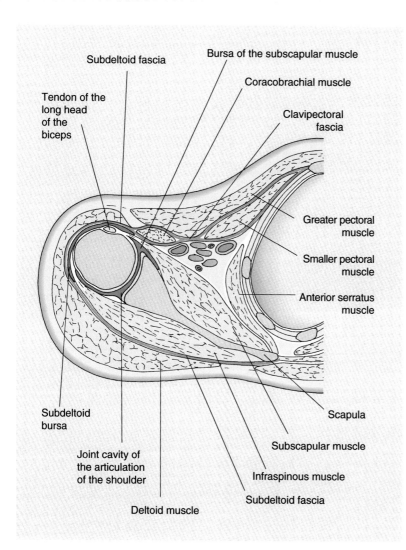

cuff of the pectoral girdle and the upper end of the humerus. It is particularly important because of its contact with the elements of the circulatory and nervous system at the transition between the shoulder and upper arm. In a horizontal cross-section, this disk of connective tissue displays a slightly arched triangular shape. If we localize the course of the nerves and blood vessels within this triangular shape, it is easy to see what a limiting effect the forces of contraction have on the passage of nerves and blood vessels and therefore on the blood supply and nerve function.

In addition to the layers mentioned above, there are numerous other elements of the fascial network that influence the shoulder joint and its movement function. Because of their particular significance, I would like to emphasize the serratus anterior muscle, the levator scapulae, and their fasciae. However, sheet-like layers such as the trapezius and latissimus dorsi muscles can play a role in a dysfunction of the shoulder joint as well. It is a characteristic of the fascial network that it cannot be forced into one general pattern; there are always special individual forms. However, one fundamental rule is repeatedly shown to be true: the portions of the fascial network that are connected to small muscular units or muscles that have only a limited range of flexion and extension are more significant for the stability of bodily form than those aspects of the fascial network that surround muscles with a very large area.

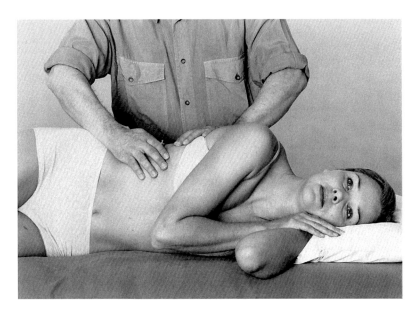

Figure 4.61 Examination of the connection between the external oblique and the serratus anterior.

The techniques described above follow this fundamental rule. For this reason, they are primarily focused on the fasciae of the pectoralis minor, infraspinatus, supraspinatus, and subclavius muscles so that a maximally stable treatment result may be guaranteed with a minimum of treatment.

Examination of the shoulder region

In order to evaluate a dysfunction of the shoulder joint in the context of the overall structure, it is helpful to first observe the patient's usual sequence of movement. This observation gives us an insight into the everyday posture into which a dysfunction of this joint is integrated.

First, watch the patient from one side, both sitting and standing.

Pay attention to the spatial relationship between the hip axis and the shoulder. If the shoulder appears to be slouched forward relative to the hip axis, i.e. if it droops strongly forward over the ribcage, this is a sign of a lack of movement coordination in the region of the serratus anterior muscle. In this case, it is valuable to examine the patient while the patient is lying on one side and pay particular attention to the connection area between the external oblique muscle and the serratus anterior (see Fig. 4.60). A lack of activity by the serratus anterior is frequently responsible for the thorax sinking down in the posterior direction along the lateral line. In such a case, the connection between the external oblique and the serratus anterior will feel rigid. The interdigitating border between the two muscles is sensitive to pressure and can be moved only a small distance relative to the ribs located below it, and the associated fasciae appear fibrous.

In a second step of the examination, compare the normal position of both shoulders from the front and from behind to see how they connect into the ribcage and the arms. Ask the patient to raise both arms and observe this motion from the side. Continue the examination by passively guiding the motion of one arm at a time in order to identify local limitations associated with the coordinative level of movement.

In order to include patterns of ligamentous tension in our observations, we should also examine the sternoclavicular joint. Because patients virtually never feel symptomatic pain in the region of this joint and, in my experience, want the therapist to treat the painful shoulder directly, it is easy for us to overlook the significance of the sternoclavicular joint.[2]

_____

[2] The test for the sternoclavicular joint is described in detail in Barral _et al._ (1993: 70).

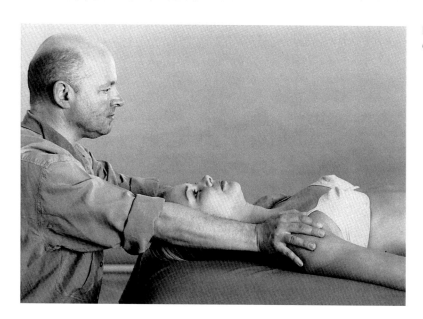

Figure 4.62   Shoulder test in the dorsal position.

Besides the ligamentous components, the subclavius muscle, with its strongly pronounced fascia, is also responsible for the fixation of the sternoclavicular joint. This muscle connects the clavicle to the first rib. It plays a decisive role in venous return from the neck region to the extent that the subclavius vein runs between the anterior scalene muscle and the subclavius muscle. As so often occurs in places of transition, a restriction of movement means not only a reduction in motor function, but also a change in fluid exchange, in this case the venous return.

A similar pattern may be found in the case of nerve supply. The course of the brachial plexus at the level of the clavicle is structured as a sliding passage surrounded by fatty and connective tissue. Like the venous passage, it can tolerate only a limited level of stabilizing pressure. If the surrounding fatty and connective tissue of the nerve is subjected to too much pressure, it will no longer be able to adapt to the abduction movement of the upper arm. Thus, the tension and pressure conditions are altered in the sheath layers of individual nerve fibers. This process affects not only the transitional passage between the shoulder and upper arm, but potentially other important bottlenecks of the nerve located farther below: in the elbow joint and carpal tunnel as well as Guyon's canal. Because of the comprehensive significance of the subclavius muscle

and its fascia, a precise examination is recommended for any dysfunction in the pectoral region.

Shoulder test in the dorsal position

Patient   Supine, both legs extended, arms resting beside the torso.

Therapist   Sitting at the head.

Contact   With the palms over the shoulder joints.

Action   The therapist pushes the shoulder elastically in the inferior direction. If it is not possible to push the shoulder elastically against the ribcage, this is a sign that strong contracting forces are prevalent between the first rib and the clavicle. In order to ascertain whether the subclavius muscle and its fascia are responsible for these forces, Barral's supplementary test is recommended.

Shoulder test lying on one side according to Barral

Patient   Lying on one side, legs slightly flexed, arms in front of the torso.

Therapist   Standing behind the patient at the level of the ribcage.

Contact   With one hand in the lateral region of the deltoid muscle, with the thumb, index finger,

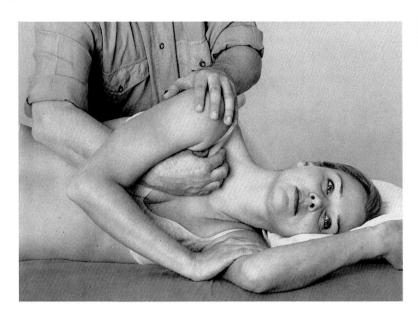

Figure 4.63 Shoulder test lying on one side according to Barral.

and middle finger of the other hand surrounding the clavicle.

Action The therapist reaches below the upper arm of the patient and surrounds the clavicle from below with the thumb and from above with the index and middle fingers. It is best if the contact is somewhat medial of the subclavian artery, as if to surround the clavicle. Naturally, it is not possible to surround the bone entirely, so our thumb is touching the two fingers only in our imagination. The contact is strong and yet slightly elastic. With the other hand, the therapist then surrounds the shoulder from behind and examines whether it can be pushed upward and forward. Normally, the subclavius muscle would yield for such a movement; however, long-term tension around the subclavius muscle and its fascia will resist this movement.

Before we decide on a treatment technique for the shoulder, it is necessary to take another look at the larger fascial context. If the restriction of movement in the joint arose from a mechanical shock to the shoulder, the local technique has a good chance of success. In this case, an overstretching of individual fiber groups occurs in the ligaments near the joint. The ligaments are no longer able to clearly perform their orienting function for muscular activity, and a typical restriction of movement occurs when the upper arm is raised or moved backwards.

However, we sometimes encounter a periarthritis of the joint without a mechanical trauma having occurred. In these cases, it is valuable to examine the transition between the abdominal cavity and ribcage precisely. Barral pointed out that a significant interdependency exists between the restriction of the costal and vertebral joints on the one hand and the restrictions of movement of the liver on the other hand. He assumes that tensions in the region of the sheath layer of the liver are transmitted throughout the fascial system and usually to the right shoulder (Barral and Mercier 2002: 100–1).

We can only guess how this transmission of tension occurs. It is possible that there is a transmission of fascial tension, because an interdependence appears to exist between the restrictions of individual costal vertebral joints and the liver, and in this manner, producing an irritation of the cervical and brachial plexus (Barral and Mercier 2002: 101–2).

Interestingly, a comparable relationship can be observed in the region of the left shoulder; here though, it is to dysfunctions of the stomach that periarthritis can be attributed (Barral 2002: 74).

Our practical experience confirms Barral's assumption. It seems that periarthritis of the joints of the pectoral girdle occurs far more frequently in the context of organ dysfunction than through mechanical trauma to a joint. For this reason, it is advisable to supplement examination of the joint in functional disorders of the shoulder with examination of the upper abdominal organs using Barral's inhibition tests.[3]

Treatment techniques

Treatment of the fascia of the pectoralis minor in relation to the fascial investment of the latissimus dorsi muscle

Patient   Seated, hip axis slightly higher than the knees.

Therapist   Seated next to the patient.

Contact   With one thumb in the front region of the axilla, with the second thumb in the rear region of the axilla, while the palms support the upper chest region from the front and the scapula from the rear.

Action   First, the therapist raises the patient's shoulder somewhat and moves the thumb in the rear region of the axilla around the common fascial investment of the latissimus dorsi muscle and the teres major muscle in order to create a firm contact point there. Using the palm, the therapist guides the shoulder slightly forward and then makes contact in an analogous fashion with the fascia of the pectoralis minor and teres minor muscles. To a certain degree, the shoulder is now riding on the therapist's two thumbs. In a second step, the thumbs follow the shoulder with "listening." If the shoulder moves forward, the therapist follows

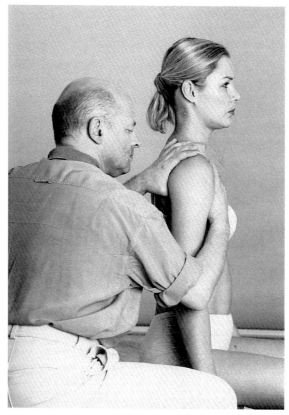

Figure 4.64   Treatment of the fascia of the pectoralis minor in relation to the fascial investment of the latissimus dorsi muscle.

this movement with both hands and intensifies this movement somewhat until it comes to a stop. At the same moment, the therapist intensifies the contact with the fascia of the pectoralis minor and teres minor muscles and exerts an active stretching impulse so as to continue following the shoulder with "listening." The shoulder will now move backwards somewhat. The therapist follows this movement until the contact in the rear region of the axilla intensifies. The therapist exerts gentle pressure on the fascia of the latissimus dorsi and teres major muscle. This entire sequence of movements can be repeated three to four times. If the shoulder slips backwards at the beginning of "listening," we first follow this movement and then exert a stretching impulse at the endpoint in the rear axilla so as to follow it forward and perform a more gentle correction there as well.

[3] Barral (2002: 14): "One hand rotates the arm in an abduction–adduction pattern and the other hand sets a visceral inhibition point. Let us assume that you suspect the possible involvement of the liver in a case of periarthritis on the right side. After you have abducted the right arm and rotated it outward, lift the liver slightly […]. If this allows you to attain an increase in mobility of at least 20 percent, you can assume that the cause of the shoulder problem lies either in the liver or the right kidney that is connected to the liver."

The patient should keep the shoulder region as relaxed as possible during this entire technique and the therapist should select the quality of the touch so as to guide the movement of the shoulder without inducing an increased muscle tone. As soon as the patient moves the shoulder actively, it is no longer possible to reach sufficiently deeply into the axilla. The goal of this treatment concept is to allow the shoulder to ride passively on the ribcage, follow the "listening," and to provide a clear, corrective impulse in the fascial system at the end of each "listening." This impulse may be strong, but should reach carefully through the fascial layers located farther outward without injuring them.

Treatment of the fascia infraspinata

Patient   Supine, both knees flexed.

Therapist   Sitting next to the treatment table.

Contact   With the fingertips of one hand directly on the fascia infraspinata while the other hand surrounds the shoulder to provide support.

Action   The therapist accepts the weight of the shoulder by raising it imperceptibly. Then the fingertips carefully reach through the skin and superficial fascia so as to come into strong contact with the fascia infraspinata. For this type of contact, it is important to bear in mind that the fascia infraspinata contains aponeurotic elements. The fascia should be touched as if we were reaching through the tissue to the attachment to the bone. The touch will become particularly effective in the boundary layers between aponeurotic elements and less fibrous fascial layers. These boundary layers may have very different individual courses. It is necessary to localize them precisely before we influence the fascia directly. In contrast to the treatment of the fascia of the pectoralis minor, this is a purely direct technique. We act directly on the connection of the aponeurotic layer to the adjacent regions by maintaining the strong contact with the fingertips during a minimal sliding motion. We must pay particular attention to the points that overlap with other fasciae:

- in the medial direction, the fascia of the rhomboid muscle

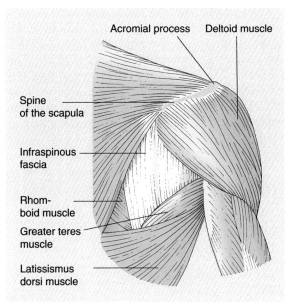

Figure 4.65   Course of the fascia infraspinata in relation to the adjacent muscles.

- in the lateral direction, the fascia of the deltoid muscle
- in the inferior direction, the fascial investment of the latissimus dorsi and teres major muscles.

Treatment of the fascia of the subclavius muscle

Patient   Prone, the shoulder to be treated resting on the edge of the treatment table while the arm hangs off to the side

Therapist   Sitting at the level of the patient's shoulder

Contact   With flexed fingertips in the fascial space below the clavicle while the other hand guides the patient's hanging arm.

Action   The therapist surrounds the subclavius muscle from below at the point at which its fascia comes into contact with the extensions of the serratus anterior and the external intercostal muscles.

The fingertips gradually come into stronger contact with the fascial investment of the muscle without touching the nearby vessels. It is best for this contact to be made by the patient gradually allowing the weight of the upper thoracic region to sink into the therapist's hand. At the same time, the therapist's other hand carefully guides the

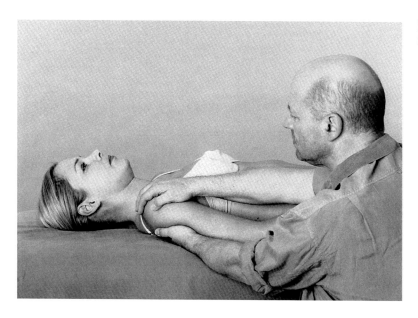

Figure 4.66   Treatment of the fascia infraspinata.

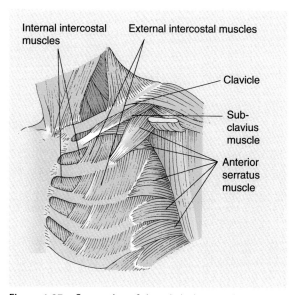

Figure 4.67   Connection of the subclavius muscle, serratus anterior and external intercostal muscles.

patient's upper arm upward, almost to the level of the treatment table. This movement may only continue as long as no resistance is encountered. Subsequently, the therapist pushes the upper arm into the joint with gently elastic pressure. A shear force occurs along the muscle fibers of the subclavius muscle, which continues through the clavicle into the sternoclavicular joint. By gently turning the upper arm and altering the angle of

the upper arm and pectoral girdle, it is now possible to reach different layers of fascia.

> We can increase the efficacy of this technique by including the muscular activity of the serratus anterior. For this purpose, we must raise the patient's upper arm a little more in relation to the ribcage and ask the patient to use the arm to push against our pressure. However, the use of the patient's muscular activity in a problem-free manner is possible only if no drastic restriction of movement is present. In my experience, it is more effective to treat a pronounced impingement with passive movement. In my practice, Barral's procedure has been shown to be effective (see below).

Barral's treatment of the subclavius muscle

Patient   Lying on one side, knee slightly flexed.

Therapist   Standing behind the patient.

Contact   With the index and middle fingers on one hand above the clavicle and the thumb below it, while the other hand surrounds the shoulder from behind.

Action   With the index and middle fingers from above and with the thumb from below, the therapist

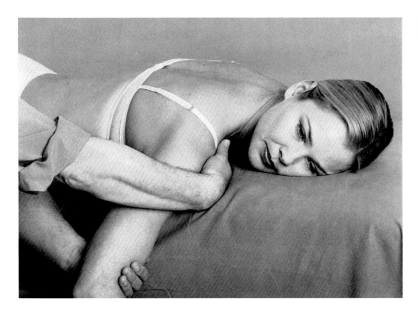

Figure 4.68 Treatment of the fascia of the subclavius muscle.

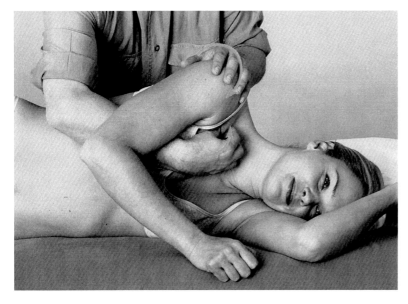

Figure 4.69 Barral's treatment of the subclavius muscle.

grasps the clavicle in an approximately medial direction from the course of the subclavian artery, as if to surround the clavicle. While maintaining this contact, the therapist pushes the shoulder in a circular motion upward, forward, and then downward and finally describes a complete circle back to the initial position. While doing so, the therapist is looking for any resistance that may be noticeable.

The efficacy of this technique succeeds or fails with the sensitivity of our touch: while the clavicle remains firmly surrounded, it is important to avoid

resistances with minimal avoidance maneuvers, i.e. the circular motions of the shoulder are varied. In this process, the clavicle comes to attention on the sternum like a tiny flagpole; it makes a small circular motion in the connection to the sternum while we make a larger circle with the shoulder. This gives us the ability to affect the ligamentary tensions of the sternoclavicular joint and the muscular tension patterns and the fascial tension of the subclavius muscle and all of the muscles that participate in shoulder motions at the same time.

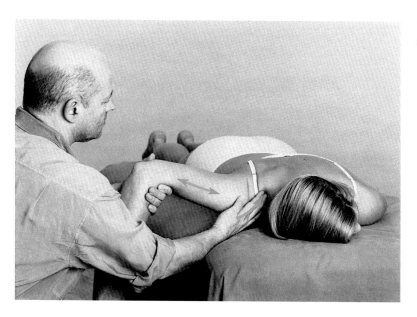

Figure 4.70   Treatment of the fascia supraspinata.

Treatment of the fascia supraspinata

Patient   Prone.

Therapist   Sitting at the level of the pectoral girdle.

Contact   With the fingertips of one hand reaching through the superficial layers of the trapezius muscle.

Action   Similar to the preceding treatment of the sheath layer of the subclavius muscle, the clavipectoral fascia, the therapist abducts the patient's arm and lifts it. If a resistance to movement occurs, it is important to avoid the restriction by using minimal movements. At the same time, we use the fingers of the other hand to reach through the superficial layers until we feel the tension of the supraspinatus muscle. It is now crucial that we direct our attention to the prominence of individual groups of fasciae. As soon as we observe a high-density group of fibers, we gradually intensify our contact at this point. At the same time, we slide the upper arm into the joint so that the joint capsule can relax somewhat. As soon as this relaxation occurs, we modify the angle between the upper arm and the thorax minimally in various directions until a change in tone occurs at the critical point of the supraspinatus muscle. At that moment, we reduce the shear force between the upper arm and the shoulder joint by allowing the arm to follow gravity and glide slightly out of the glenoid fossa.

> Because the fascia supraspinata is closely connected to the coracoacromial ligament, we should make a constant effort during treatment to ensure that as regulatory an effect as possible occurs on this ligament as well. In a joint that offers as much range of motion as the shoulder joint, we should avoid pulling the fascia apart mechanically. The goal is to provide a sustained impulse on the critical bundle of fasciae and, at the same time, to observe the effects on the ligaments near the joint.

Treatment of the fascia infraspinata and the fascia supraspinata

Patient   Lying supine, both knees flexed so that the soles of both feet are in complete contact with the treatment table.

Therapist   Sitting below the pectoral girdle.

Contact   With both palms and the fingertips of both hands.

Action   The therapist first abducts the patient's arm and guides it into elevation. In this starting

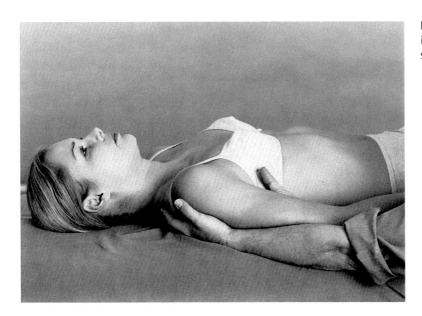

Figure 4.71   Treatment of the fascia infraspinata and the fascia supraspinata.

position, the therapist's forearm supports the patient's upper arm. The second support surface is provided by the palm on the upper third of the scapula. This double support is necessary in order to have both hands free for direct contact with the fascial layers of the infraspinatus and supraspinatus muscles. While the supporting contact in maintained, the therapist's fingertips reach strongly into the fascia infraspinata and the fingertips of the other hand reach through the layer of the trapezius muscle at the point where the coracoacromial ligament is embedded in the fascia supraspinata. In this manner, the scapula and clavicle are resting in their fascial bed in such a way that they will be able to tilt relative to one another in three-dimensional space. While we, figuratively speaking, make both bones hover in their fascial suspension, we now give a gentle push on the joint capsule with both support surfaces, i.e. we move our forearm, which is supporting the patient's upper arm, and our palm, which is holding the scapula, very slightly toward one another. As soon as a counterpressure occurs, we follow it and guide the arm minimally out of the joint. With some skill, we can evoke an indirect relaxation of the fibers that connect directly to the joint capsule. During this process, we intensify the contact between our fingertips and the fasciae infraspinata and supraspinata. In other words, we are working indirectly and with detailed "listening"

in the interior of the joint while, at the same time, we exert a direct and very drastic influence on both of the decisive fasciae.

The efficiency of this method lies in the fact that the subtle, indirect access of the joint capsule is combined with a very direct treatment of both fasciae (infraspinata and supraspinata). The patient's arm should be elevated only as far as is possible without causing pain. In the case of a drastic restriction of movement, it is advisable to abduct the arm only to a small extent and guide it very slightly upward during treatment in minimal passive movement steps. It is a considerable technical challenge for the therapist to conduct two fundamentally different modes of treatment with the same hand and arm.

Additional remarks

At the beginning of this chapter, I mentioned that the shoulder joint is described in the literature as the most mobile of all the joints. In local treatment, this mobility requires a considerable amount of precision. Imprecise influence on the fascial sheath of the joint may encourage momentary changes in tension, but may also destabilize the joint under certain circumstances. For this reason, the precision of the manual influence on fasciae in the immediate vicinity of the joint has essential significance if the treatment is to have a lasting result.

However, in addition to the need for precise, detailed work of correction, there is also a global context of bodily form within which the joint is arranged. The manner in which the thorax as a whole rests on the organ column of the abdominal cavity, the spatial relationship of the hip axis and pectoral girdle, and also the preferred movement patterns of the arms and hands, are all reflected in the fascial network. The quality of the the client's movements allows the therapist to read how the individual segments of the torso are connected. Under certain circumstances, the problem zone of the shoulders is merely a response to structural weaknesses in a deeper zone of transition. This is primarily true in the case of the transition between the abdominal cavity and chest cavity.

I have already mentioned Barral's hypothesis regarding the relationship between the shoulder joint and restrictions of movement in the organs located below the diaphragm, and this is certainly very significant. Moreover, there are many other critical zones within the fascial system whose tension patterns have an influence that reaches into the shoulders. Because the pectoral girdle is located between the relatively immobile ribcage and the neck region, which is mobile, it must be able to adapt to the dynamic rotational forces acting from the cranial direction as well as the shear forces acting from the base below it. In my opinion, it is for this reason that the treatment of restrictions of movement at the transition between the abdominal and chest cavities is sometimes not entirely sufficient to guarantee a stable result. It is wise also to examine and treat the transitions between the individual curvatures of the back. We must direct our attention to how the curve of the sacrum meets the lumbar region, how the upper lumbar spine is connected to the thoracic region, and how the uppermost section of the back transitions into the neck. Correspondingly, we encounter a small selection of techniques for the treatment of the pectoral girdle before we begin the detail corrections on the shoulder joint itself. In practice it has proved useful first to treat the transitions between the curvatures of

the back and the transitions between visceral cavities before a precise treatment of the shoulder joint.

4.4   UPPER EXTREMITY: UPPER ARM, FOREARM, AND HAND

Aspects of form

The fasciae of the arms are subjected to different functional demands from the fasciae of the pectoral girdle. The influence of gravity on the pectoral girdle is cushioned by a dynamic visceral cavity and the curvatures of the back. Such a dynamic is lacking within the arm: there is no buffer within this extremity like the visceral cavity, while the respiratory motion acts only as a minimal rotational force on the tissue without causing a significant change in the position of the arm. Let us regard these circumstances in relation to our central working hypothesis, which is that fasciae and membranes change their appearance according to their functional context. As soon as repetitive sequences of movement occur, the fibers realign themselves correspondingly and regulate the distribution of components with high and low fluid contents. The dominant functions of the arms are flexion and extension and the interplay between those two functions. This is clearly reflected in the layers of the fasciae of the upper arm and forearm. Here, there are none of the flat sliding layers as can be found in the pectoral girdle. Instead, there are deep membranes that form individual osteofibrous canals for flexors and extensors, respectively.

In most day-to-day activities, the flexion movement of the forearm and the extension movement of the hand are dominant. So, in people who perform a manual activity, we usually find a lack of equilibrium in the joints of the arm between the prevailing tone of the flexors and the tone of the extensors. The resting tension of the flexors is elevated in comparison with the resting tension of the extensors. The fasciae of the flexor musculature are subjected to different forces than those of the extensor musculature. Because these fasciae have a direct connection to the intermuscular septa and interosseus membranes, this lack of equilibrium between flexors and extensors also has an effect within the membrane structure of the osteofibrous canals. In my opinion, the

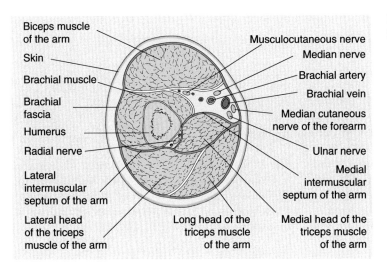

Biceps muscle of the arm
Skin
Brachial muscle
Brachial fascia
Humerus
Radial nerve
Lateral intermuscular septum of the arm
Lateral head of the triceps muscle of the arm
Long head of the triceps muscle of the arm
Musculocutaneous nerve
Median nerve
Brachial artery
Brachial vein
Median cutaneous nerve of the forearm
Ulnar nerve
Medial intermuscular septum of the arm
Medial head of the triceps muscle of the arm

Figure 4.72   Cross-section at the level of the middle of the upper arm.

limits that we encounter in the treatment of muscular function of the arms may be traced back to this fact. At some point, the lack of equilibrium between the tone of the flexor and extensor musculature is present not only in the fascial layer of the arm, but also in the deep membranes. In advanced stages, the deep membranes have a higher fiber density and fewer elastic components than the superficial layers, which can no longer be solved with muscle-building and equalizing activity. Faced with this situation, we must rely on a detailed treatment strategy that allows the musculature to gain a new range of action by treating the deep membrane layers.

Anatomy of the fasciae and membranes

The fascial sheath of the upper arm, the brachial fascia, surrounds the entire upper arm. Its layers are more strongly pronounced on the lateral and dorsal sides of the arm. Strangely, this fascial layer is present on the strong flexor of the upper arm, the biceps brachii muscle, only as a delicate, thin layer. The fibers of the brachial fascia primarily run perpendicular to the fiber path of the musculature it encloses. The fascia transitions seamlessly into the adjacent fasciae: distally into the antebrachial fascia and proximally into the axillary fascia and the fasciae of the pectoral girdle.

It is a characteristic of the fasciae of the extremities that they serve as both a superficial sheath as well as a partition separating antagonistic muscle groups internally within the limbs, that is, as intermuscular septa. Thus, delicate dividing layers extend from the antebrachial fascia to the periosteum of the humerus. These dividing layers, the medial septum and lateral septum, divide the upper arm into two self-contained chambers in which the flexion musculature runs on the ventral side and the extensor musculature runs on the dorsal side.

The medial intermuscular septum runs between the attachment of the coracobrachialis muscle and the medial epicondyle. The less strongly pronounced lateral intermuscular septum extends between the attachment of the deltoid muscle and the lateral epicondyle.

Both intermuscular septa serve as muscular attachments, the medial septum as an origin for the fibers of the brachialis and the medial head of the triceps brachii, the lateral septum for the fibers of the triceps brachii, the brachialis, the brachioradialis, and the extensor carpi radialis longus.

For manual treatment techniques, it is important to keep in mind that the brachial fascia surrounds the surface of the arm, but is also responsible for the deep structure. According to observations in practice, it is not possible to treat one layer without producing an effect on the other.

I have already mentioned that the brachial fascia of the upper arm transitions seamlessly into the antebrachial fascia of the forearm. Using the example of this fascia, it is possible to clearly see how

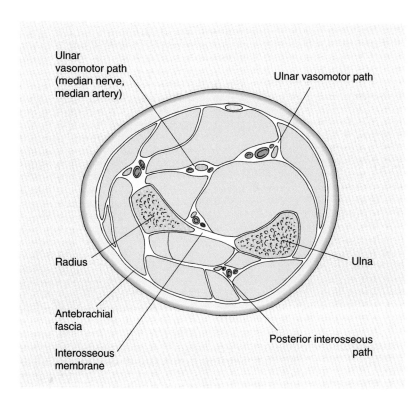

Figure 4.73 Fascial chambers at the level of the middle of the forearm in cross-section.

Ulnar vasomotor path (median nerve, median artery)

Ulnar vasomotor path

Radius

Ulna

Antebrachial fascia

Posterior interosseous path

Interosseous membrane

unilateral pressure and tension forces change the texture of the connective tissue. It is not for nothing that the forearm and the transition to the hand are particularly susceptible to a phenomenon that has recently gained increased attention as *repetitive stress syndrome* or *repetitive strain syndrome*.

The kinds of strain to which the forearms and hands are subjected are so variable that we must always take into account the idiosyncratic form of their connective tissues. With high levels of strain, the proximal layers of the antebrachial fascia can become very dense, almost aponeurotic. The density of the fibers is particularly palpable at the transition to the wrist, specifically in the area in which the fasciae are aligned in a circular shape parallel to one another and condense as the flexor retinaculum. It is important for treatment practice to bear in mind that this band does not maintain its tension pattern independently from the global fascial tension of the forearm. The chances of treatment are very favorable when the dense fibers of the flexor retinaculum ligament (also called the transverse carpal ligament) are embedded in an environment of antebrachial fascia that is generally tense.

The transition between the forearm and hand as a critical zone plays an important role, in particular for nerve supply. The transition between the upper arm and forearm is similar. There as well, in the case of repetitive muscle activity, we encounter tough layers that can place the nerve passages under pressure. The bicipital aponeurosis plays an essential role here as a bridge that may reduce space because, as a fibrous extension of the bicipital fasciae, which are weakly pronounced in and of themselves, it fixes sustained bending tendencies at the elbow joint.

The fascia of the forearm is closely connected to the periosteum of the edge of the ulna and to the distal third of the radius and, with its dividing layers, reaches into the deep layers of the forearm. In treatment practice, the close connection to the bones of the forearm allows us indirect access to the interior membrane connections of both bones. In my opinion, the attachment of the fascia of the forearm to the posterior edge of the ulna allows us a highly efficient access to the entire tension complex of the elbow joint. Similarly to the upper arm, we find the manifestation of functionally bundled chambers in

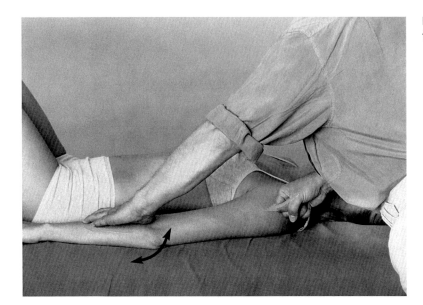

Figure 4.74 Treatment of the deep fascial layer according to Ida Rolf.

the forearm as well: fascial dividing walls separate and contain antagonistic groups of muscles.

The deepest dividing layer between flexors and extensors of the forearm is the antebrachial interosseus membrane. Like the interosseus membrane of the lower leg, it plays the deciding role in securing the bones against lateral displacement. In my opinion, the treatment of this membrane plays a prominent role among the techniques for the upper extremity (see below, under Treatment techniques).

If we continue to follow the course of the forearm fascia in the distal direction, we encounter a distinct difference between the flexor and extensor side of the hand: the fasciae of the back of the hand, the extensor side, have a relatively delicate structure and play a subordinate role in treatment. In contrast, the fasciae of the flexor side are complex and very fibrous in some levels. Directly under the surface of the hand, we find the flat palmar aponeurosis, which is a direct extension of the fascia of the forearm and, on the muscular level, represents an extension of the palmaris longus. It connects the fascia of the forearm to the four fingers. Shortly before its intersection with the finger joints, it is reinforced with transverse bundles of fibers, the transverse fasciculi.

In the deeper layers of the hand, the fasciae form individual chambers for the tendons. Here, these fascial dividing walls are more or less perpendicular

to the palmar fascia of the palm located above them; in the direction of the deepest flexor layer, they are also perpendicular to a thinly pronounced fascial layer.

Treatment techniques

Treatment of the deep fascial layer according to Ida Rolf

To a large extent, Ida Rolf's technique for the treatment of the deep fascia in the region of the upper extremity acts parallel to the path of the muscle fibers and transverse to the fiber direction of the fascia. It is characteristic for this treatment that the therapist uses the patient's active joint movement to assist the technique and is thus able to facilitate a deep effect for a technique that is applied to the surface.

Patient   Supine, both legs flexed, arms next to the torso.

Therapist   Standing at the level of the patient's pectoral girdle.

Contact   With the surface of the first phalanges of the fingers of a gently closed fist at the level of the deltoid muscle and, with the other hand, direct with the antebrachial fascia.

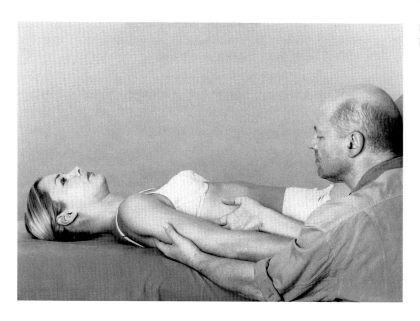

Figure 4.75 Treatment of the intermuscular septa of the upper arm.

Action We act on the fascia at both contact points in such a way that we cross the fibers with strong pressure. In so doing we slide over the exterior surrounding layer extremely slowly and ensure that the pressure is exerted not directly onto the deep layers, but rather diagonally onto the bone. While we maintain this slowly gliding contact, we ask the patient to move the elbow joint approximately 2 cm outward and inward several times.

> The amount of pressure used should be in relation to the fascial tone of the layers being treated. We should not exert any pressure from our shoulder joint, but rather successively relocate our weight into both of our hands. The patient's elbow movement allows us to achieve an effect on the intermuscular septa.

Treatment of the intermuscular septa of the upper arm

Patient Supine, both legs flexed, arms resting next to the torso.

Therapist Sitting to the side at the level of the upper abdominal cavity.

Contact With the fingertips of one hand at the connection between the medial brachial intermuscular septum and the periosteum of the upper arm, with the fingertips of the other hand on the connection between the lateral septum and the periosteum of the upper arm.

Action With the fingertips of both hands, we carefully feel our way to the point where the medial brachial intermuscular septum transitions into the periosteum of the upper arm. At the same time, we use the fingertips of our other hand to create contact with the transitional point of the lateral septum on the bone. In so doing, we should carefully avoid the fatty and connective tissue bed of the nerves and blood vessels, produce a very energetic contact, and act directly on the connection between the septa and the periosteum.

> Direct influence on the dividing layers between the flexors and extensors of the upper arm takes place as if we were trying to loosen the tissue of the triceps muscle from the bone. This active stretching should be combined with "listening" because the septa respond to overly direct influence with resistance. Attentiveness is also required for the radial nerve. Pushing the radial nerve and its adjacent blood vessels against the humerus from behind would have an adverse effect on the treatment.

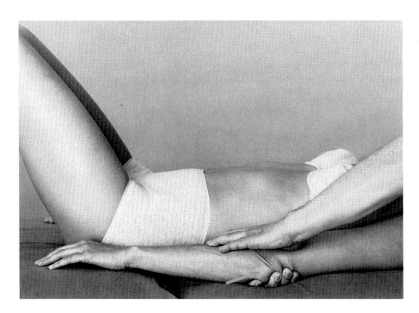

Figure 4.76   Treatment of the antebrachial fascia according to Ida Rolf.

Treatment of the antebrachial fascia according to Ida Rolf

Patient   Lying supine, both legs flexed, arms resting next to the torso.

Therapist   Standing at the level of the patient's upper arm.

Contact   With the fingertips of one hand below the medial epicondyle and surrounding the medial edge of the ulna. At the same time, with the fingertips of the other hand alternating on the surrounding fascial layer of various extensors.

Action   We surround the ulna from the medial direction by reaching through the fascia of the forearm and the aponeurosis of the biceps brachii into the flexor carpi ulnaris. Figuratively speaking, we anchor our fingertips deep in the tissue like a flexible hook. With our other hand, we also use our fingertips to make contact with the layer of fascia surrounding the level of the midsection of the brachioradialis. While we are then pushing the tissue of the ulna, i.e. the flexors in the elbow joint, strongly in the cranial direction, we stretch the fascial layer of the extensors farther into extension. While the contact in the region of the flexors remains the same, the strong contact in the region of the extensors ranges from the brachioradialis to the extensor carpi radialis longus and brevis.

In order to achieve a truly three-dimensional deep effect on the fascial network in the entire area of the forearm, it is helpful to enlist the aid of the flexion and extension movements. While we maintain an "anchor" point in the flexors and actively stretch the layers of the extensors, we ask the patient first to extend the hand flatly along the treatment surface, then to stretch the fingers up toward the ceiling, and finally to allow the hand to follow the fingers in the stretch. In the countermovement, the palm returns first from the extension and then the fingers follow. Then we ask the patient to slowly make a fist and then open the fist again.

The patient's active movement allows us access to very different areas of the fascial network. In so doing, we take into account that there are three fascial chambers in the forearm: one for the ventral muscle group of the extensors, one for the dorsal group of the flexors, and finally one for the group that is displaced in the ventral direction and innervated by the radial nerve, and which has an intermediate position between the flexors and extensors. Contact by the therapist with both hands is strongly maintained on the flexor side, while the therapist's fingertips very slowly slide in the fascia of the extensors.

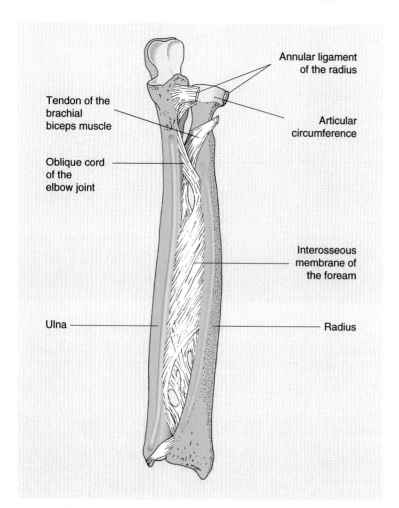

Tendon of the brachial biceps muscle

Oblique cord of the elbow joint

Ulna

Annular ligament of the radius

Articular circumference

Interosseous membrane of the foream

Radius

Figure 4.77   Interosseous membranes of the forearm, with the annular ligament in cross-section.

Treatment of the interosseous membrane of the forearm

Patient   Lying supine, legs flexed, arms resting next to the torso.

Therapist   Standing at the level of the patient's pectoral girdle.

Contact   With the surface of the second phalanx of the index and middle fingers of one hand, while the other hand supports the forearm from behind.

Action   Like the treatment technique described above, it is important here as well to surround the forearm from below and press it against the upper arm in order to ensure that the joint capsule relaxes during the application of pressure. With the other hand, we apply gradually increasing pressure in the direction of the interosseus membrane (using either our fingertips or, in the case of strongly pronounced musculature, the second phalanges of the index and middle fingers). It is essential to the efficacy of this technique that we pay precise attention to the direction of the pressure we apply. The membrane has a hiatus in its upper portion for the radial tuberosity and the bicipital tendon that is attached there. Both bones of the forearm are stabilized against lateral displacement next to this hiatus by the strong fiber tension of the oblique cord of the elbow joint. We must now ensure that the direction of the fibers is different in this oblique cord and the substantially flatter main portion of the membrane (see Fig. 4.77). Only in the last fifth of the membrane, i.e. slightly above the wrist, is the orientation of the fibers once again parallel to that of the oblique cord.

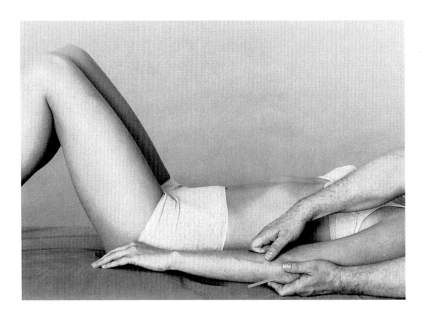

Figure 4.78 Treatment of the interosseous membrane of the forearm.

Increased tension in the region of the oblique cord can be recognized by the fact that it is no longer possible to compress elastically the ulna and radius at this point. It is important to stabilize the tissue layers that are located directly distal to the elbow joint while we work our way layer by layer through the extensors with the pressure of our fingers in the direction of the oblique cord so that we can very slowly exert an impulse there between the two bones. The pressure should work diagonally between the ulna and radius, i.e. parallel to the fiber orientation of the cord.

In the farther path of the forearm, we maintain the diagonal pressure as if we were trying to rotate the ulna toward the radius. With some practice, it is possible to apply "listening" to the membrane even during this extremely intense application of pressure. Thus, we are able to connect our direct influence to the membrane's self-regulating ability.

Treatment of the fasciae and the deep fascial chambers on the flexor side of the hand

Patient   Supine, both legs flexed, arms next to the body, the hand to be treated is resting in the therapist's hands.

Therapist   Sitting on the treatment table next to the patient.

Contact   With the flexed fingers of both hands on the medial and lateral boundary of the palmar aponeurosis.

Action   The patient positions the forearm vertically while the upper arm rests on the treatment table in the shoulder region. The therapist now surrounds the layers distally from the flexor ligament slightly laterally and medially from the palmar aponeurosis, applies pressure to the tissue, and follows the effect of this pressure with "listening." The patient's hand initially remains flexed. The therapist now gradually begins to change the position of the wrist in space and, while doing so, combines the subtly stretching of the fascia with passive pronation and supination. Owing to the change in the tension conditions, "listening" now provides information about the deep fascial chambers of the hand. It is important to give a sustained impulse only where the most distinct compression of tissue is found.

Manual treatment of the hand requires precise, detailed knowledge and a high degree of strength and sensitivity. The necessary strong contact should not be alternated with stiff pressure because the deep chambers of the fascial system respond negatively to "pulling" attempts to stretch them.

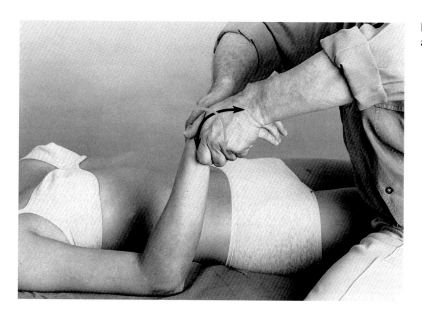

Figure 4.79   Treatment of the fasciae and deep fascial chambers of the hand.

TREATMENT OF CARPAL TUNNEL SYNDROME

Conceptual background

There are two fundamental preconditions for the undisturbed function of a nerve: the nerve requires a positive basic tension and a certain degree of mobility relative to adjacent layers, known as boundary layers. Only then is it possible for the chemical life processes of the nerve to function optimally. The basis of this process is primarily arterial oxygen supply and, in addition, its supply of transmitters and enzymes.[4]

To a large extent, the functionality of a nerve is dependent upon its oxygen supply. This supply process in turn is dependent upon a particular pressure gradient between arterial pressure and the pressure acting on the nerve from the surrounding tissue. To a certain degree, the nerve is capable of adjusting to conditions of unfavorable pressure. It has a control organ, known as the nervi nervorum. The nervi nervorum are small branches of the nerve that provide information to the central nervous system about the interior condition of the nerve and the pressure conditions on

the boundary surfaces. The nerve is able to correct the pressure conditions over the long term by forming additional fascicles and epineurial connective tissue. However, it is precisely this protective process that can damage the nerve in the passages where there is not enough room for connective tissue to absorb additional pressure. The carpal tunnel is one such passage. The carpal bones and flexor retinaculum surrounding the tunnel form a bottleneck in which even a small deposit of protective fascicles or Renaut's bodies can overload the nerve. Van den Berg (1999: 226) reports that the increase in volume by Renaut's bodies can reach up to 30 percent of the volume of a nerve.[11]

However, the change to the connective tissue in and around the nerve is not the only source of the changes in pressure conditions. As a rule, there is either already an edemic blockage due to inflammation or a cross-sectional increase in nearby tendons over a long period in time before the increased formation of connective tissue begins.

Moreover, as we will see, there is an entire range of influencing factors that are not located directly at the carpal tunnel.

Methodical considerations

For decades, carpal tunnel syndrome has been discussed in the orthopedic literature as the most

---

[4] A detailed discussion of this subject matter may be found in van den Berg (1999: 223–31).

widespread form of lesion of peripheral nerves. The anatomical units in and around the carpal tunnel itself are at the center of the traditional orthopedic viewpoint. Therefore, it is primarily the transverse carpal ligament (also called the flexor retinaculum) and the sheaths of the tendons of the flexor musculature running through the carpal tunnel that have been described for almost a century as the pivotal anatomical units for this problem. In orthopedic examination, the etiology is concentrated on the local pressure and tension events in the carpal tunnel itself. Tension patterns located farther away from the wrist are therefore brought into consideration only to the extent that they are necessary for differential diagnostic clarification.

The treatment concept introduced here is based on the methodical assumption that disrupted tension patterns in the connective tissue system originate in an overarching context. In this sense, it makes sense to classify local tension and pressure events in and around the carpal tunnel in the context of the overarching pattern. This results in a technique that does treat large-surface layers of connective tissue, the muscular fascia, septa, and interosseus membranes, but also details such as the sheath and dividing layers of the affected nerve cords.

Therefore, it is not only the tissues running through the tunnel that are at the center of the discussion, but also the tissue layers in the region of the shoulder, the upper arm, the forearm, and also the forehand on the other side of the tunnel. Correspondingly, the nerve that is decisive for the pathology, the median nerve, is considered in its entire path, from the cranial branch at the brachial plexus into its very various paths after passing through the tunnel. Accordingly, the practical treatment suggestions target not only the local events at the carpal tunnel itself, but also the larger "tissue landscape" within which the unfavorable pressure conditions of the carpal tunnel develop.

Anatomical conditions

The carpal tunnel consists of a 2- to 3-cm long passage between the bones of the wrist and the flexor retinaculum. Viewed in cross-section, the bones of the wrist appear concavely arranged. The flexor retinaculum consists of tough fibers that are connected to the radial and ulnar eminences of the wrist. On the radial side, the flexor retinaculum is connected to the tubercles of the scaphoid bone and trapezium bone and on the ulnar side to the tubercles of the pisiform bone and hamulus of the hamate bone. Under normal conditions, the carpal tunnel guarantees that the sheath-covered tendons of eight flexor muscles and the median nerve can pass through the narrow passage. Here, the flexor retinaculum functions as the "guiding band" for the tendons passing through the carpal tunnel (Rauber and Kopsch 1987: 411).

From the structure of the carpal tunnel, it can be seen that the nerve function of the median nerve can be disturbed by spatial changes in the tunnel. Such a case occurs if constant pressure is exerted from outside on the narrow passage between the forearm and hand or if the tissue layers passing through the tunnel, i.e. the eight flexor tendons with their surrounding sheaths, or the median nerve require more space than the diameter of the tunnel. In such a situation with constantly increasing pressure in the carpal tunnel, the median nerve will be the victim of the stricture because nerve tissue is less tolerant of pressure than the sheath layer of the tendons.

It is significant for evaluating the pathology and also for treatment techniques that the median nerve is a "mixed" nerve, i.e. it contains motor, sensory, and vegetative fibers. The sensory fibers have the largest portion in terms of space (Wilhelm 1987).

The nerve is composed of many fascicles in a plexus-like connection. On the exterior, it is surrounded by a connective tissue epineurium that contains a considerable amount of fat. The fascicles themselves are also surrounded by a thin perineurium, producing a septum-like division of the fascicles. Within the fascicles, the individual nerve fibers are embedded in an elastic, finely fibrous endoneurium containing capillaries (Kleinau, unpublished: 17).

In order to be able to understand the topic of the carpal tunnel from a structural viewpoint, it is important to bear in mind that there are also elements outside the tunnel that may be susceptible to dysfunction on the nervous or muscular level: the tendon of the long palmar muscle has particular significance because it ends in the aponeurosis of the palm and thus comes into connection with the flexor retinaculum. The flexor carpi ulnaris

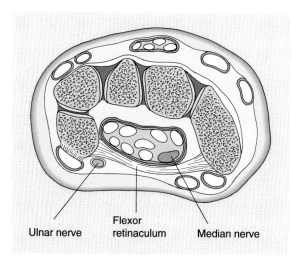

Ulnar nerve | Flexor retinaculum | Median nerve

Figure 4.80 Cross-section of the carpal tunnel.

muscle, a flexor that, with its tendon, runs outside the carpal tunnel, as well as the ulnar nerve that runs in the immediate vicinity of this muscle are important for treatment techniques as well.

From the anatomical topography of the carpal tunnel, we can gather that there are individual structural elements that, through this narrowing process, transfer increased pressure more or less directly onto the median nerve, and at a skeletal level these are primarily the hamate and capitate bones. However, any form of drastic restrictions of movement of other bones of the wrist or significant subluxations can play a role as well. At a muscular level, it is primarily the tendon sheaths adjacent to the median nerve within the carpal tunnel that are most significant for the transmission of pressure, in particular the tendon that leads to the index finger, which usually runs directly below the median nerve.

In the advanced stages of the syndrome, chief factors causing symptoms are the drastic adaptations to tissues within the carpal tunnel, which is only a few centimeters long:

- chronic fibrosis of the tendon sheaths of the flexor musculature
- various forms of edematous blockage
- demyelinization of the median nerve.

However, these changes are caused not only by physical forces and chemical metabolic processes within the tunnel; the structural basis may be found in the changes to the fascial and membrane layers that form the "tough spatial structure" of the tunnel itself. The connective tissue system is an endless system. The layers of individual types of tissue transition into one another. Therefore, purely local changes to tissue and fluid content or sliding ability of the shear lattice of collagen fibers are extraordinarily rare.

Examination

A simple test is helpful in evaluating the participation of the antebrachial fascia and interosseus membrane: we compress the forearm elastically and evaluate whether there are individual sections where there is no elastic effect.

We test the tunnel itself accordingly: is it possible to move the bones to which the flexor retinaculum is attached toward one another in such a way that the arch of the retinaculum becomes more concave? In order for this to occur, the scaphoid bone must make a slight tilting movement relative to the adjacent capitate bone. This simple test examines the "trampoline function" of the retinaculum. If no more elastic motion whatsoever results, this is a sign that the inner compression of the carpal tunnel is very advanced.

The superficial fascia and the muscular fasciae of the extremities must be differentiated structurally from the deep membranes. The treatment strategy should be selected accordingly. Superficial and muscular fasciae may be successfully treated with strong contact. When it is necessary to intensify contact, the weight of the therapist's body should be used and the therapist should avoid any tension in his or her own pectoral girdle. An elastic quality of the touch is important in order to permanently observe how the adjacent fascial layers behave during treatment. Deep membranes respond very well to "indirect maneuvers," i.e. the touch should follow the inner tensile forces of the membrane fibers up to a certain point before a correcting impulse is given.

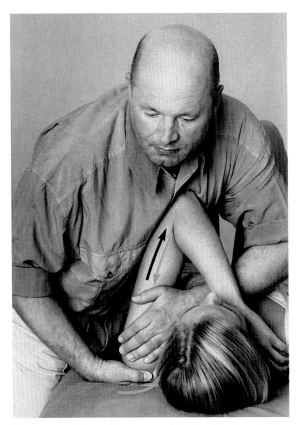

Figure 4.81   General treatment of the fascial network of the shoulder–arm connection.

Treatment technique

Step 1: Treatment of the fascial network of the shoulder–arm connection

This technique should precede an examination of the sternoclavicular joints and the upper vertebral joints of the ribs and, if necessary, a treatment of any restrictions of movement that may be localized there.[5]

Patient   Supine, both knees flexed, both arms initially resting next to the torso.

Therapist   Standing at the level of the patient's fifth rib.

---

[5] Tests for the examination of the sternoclavicular joint may be found in Barral *et al.* (1993: 69–75). Regarding the treatment techniques, see Chapter 4, Treatment of the fascia of the subclavius muscle.

Contact   One palm supports the scapula to be treated (here, the left scapula), the other hand surrounds the left shoulder joint in the region of the deltoid muscle. At the same time, using the sternum, the therapist maintains contact with the point of the elbow of the patient's raised upper arm.

Action   While the patient lies supine, the therapist uses the palm of the right hand to support the left scapula to be treated and anchors the fingertips of the same hand like a "hook" in the connection between the levator scapulae and the scapula. At the same time, the therapist's left hand surrounds the shoulder joint to be treated from above so that the acromioclavicular articulation is elastically compressed in the direction of the fiber orientation of the coracoacromial ligament. At the same time, the therapist leans from the front—coming from above with the sternum slightly against the patient's left elbow, which is pointing toward the ceiling, such that there is an elastic compression of the humerus into the shoulder. In so doing, it is important that the hand surrounding the shoulder joint stabilize the scapula and clavicle against the head of the humerus sinking into the joint. While the parts of the joint located between both hands are kept under elastic pressure, an indirect correction of relevant tissue structures is possible: the capsule is compressed, the therapist's hands move the bony parts of the joint closer together and then, following the dominant direction of tension, releases the compressed parts of the joint at the moment when a tangible counterpressure builds up. A decelerated recoil effect then occurs in the ventral part of the joint. For fans of anatomical details, the recoil effect manifests in the following ligaments: ventrally on the coracoacromial, conoid, and trapezoid ligaments and on the superior transverse ligament of the scapula; dorsally on the acromioclavicular ligament and on the posterior portion of the conoid ligament and on the superior transverse ligament of the scapula.

Step 2: Treatment of the tissue bed of the branch of the median nerve from the main nerve cord

Patient   Initial position as described in Step 1.

Therapist   Initial position as described in Step 1.

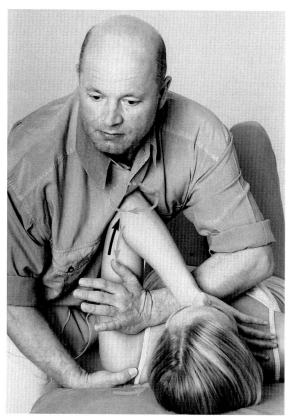

Figure 4.82   Specific treatment of the tissue bed of the branch of the median nerve from the main nerve cord.

Contact   With the palm of the right hand supporting the scapula to be treated (here, the left scapula) from the posterior side, while the pisiform bone of the left hand exerts pressure on the branch of the median nerve and the ulnar nerve of the brachial plexus from the anterior side.

Action   This time, the therapist uses his or her sternum (and therefore the patient's left elbow joint) to make a clockwise circular movement of 3 cm.

Now, in order to be able to affect the median nerve, the therapist's left hand slides very slightly downward in order to exert direct pressure from the medial side of the humerus onto the branch between the median nerve and the ulnar nerve on the brachial plexus. While the circular motion of the elbow is continued (now carefully in the counterclockwise direction as well), a passive mobilization of the tough tissue layers around the nerve occurs.

Step 3: Treatment of the transition between the upper arm and forearm with simultaneous, specific effect on the radices of the median nerve

Patient   Supine, both legs flexed, both arms resting next to the torso.

Therapist   Standing to the side at the head.

Action   The therapist's right elbow is now anchored directly at the level of the radices of the median nerve and, at the same time, the therapist surrounds the elbow joint to be treated (here, the left elbow joint) from behind. With the ring finger and middle finger of the right hand, the therapist now tries to produce as precise a contact as possible in the direction of the point at which the median nerve passes the elbow joint; this point is located precisely between the aponeurosis of the biceps brachii and the medial brachial intermuscular septum.

With the left hand, the therapist now produces a strong contact in the direction of the interosseus membrane. The pressure should be exerted diagonally between the ulna and radius and be transmitted with slow gliding centimeter by centimeter in the direction of the lower head of the radius.

Step 4: Specific effect on the passage of the median nerve in the elbow joint with simultaneous stretching effect in the carpal tunnel

Patient   Supine, both legs flexed, arms resting next to the torso.

Therapist   Standing to the side at the level of the abdomen.

Contact   With the index and middle finger of one hand at the place at which the median nerve passes the elbow joint to be treated (here, the left elbow joint), with the palm of the other hand on the tip of the elbow, while the patient's upper arm is flexed.

Action   The therapist uses the index and middle fingers to reach around the aponeurosis of the biceps while guiding the joint over the patient's head from extension into flexion in order to access the nerve as precisely as possible. The patient places the hand on the treatment table cranially of

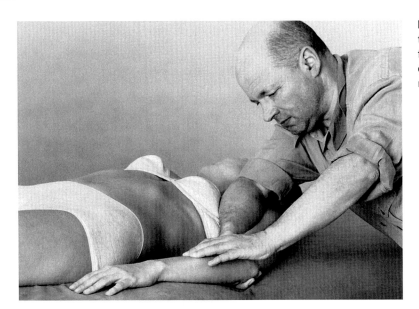

Figure 4.83   Treatment of the transition between the upper arm and forearm with simultaneous, specific effect on the radices of the median nerve.

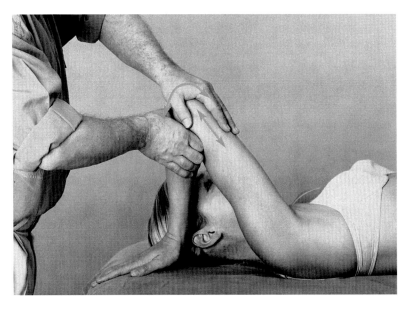

Figure 4.84   Specific effect on the passage of the median nerve in the elbow joint with simultaneous stretching effect in the carpal tunnel.

the shoulder. The patient's thumb is abducted, the contact between the hand and the treatment table is initially slightly elastic, the wrist should not be guided too far into hyperextension, especially not if there is restricted movement at a carpal bone. The therapist's left hand exerts a shear-like pressure against the elbow joint. At the same time, the therapist's other hand reaches into the interior of the elbow joint passage in order to reach the medial nerve precisely next to the path of the blood vessels, i.e. next to the aponeurosis of the biceps. If the therapist reaches somewhat higher, the ulnar nerve will be found in the direction of the triceps slightly above the medial brachial intermuscular septum; the ulnar nerve may be treated in an analogous manner. Treatment of the ulnar nerve is particularly advisable if, in addition to the carpal tunnel, a compression of the ulnar nerve has also occurred in Guyon's canal, i.e. outside of the carpal tunnel.

In both cases, in the treatment of the median nerve and of the ulnar nerve, it is essential to access the corresponding nerve as precisely as

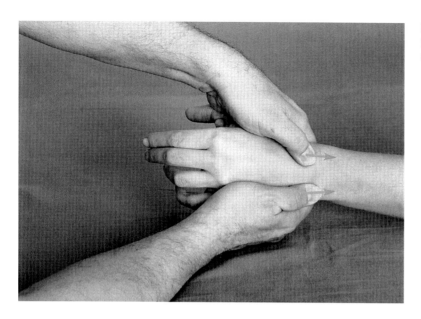

Figure 4.85   Treatment of the flexor retinaculum (from the dorsal direction).

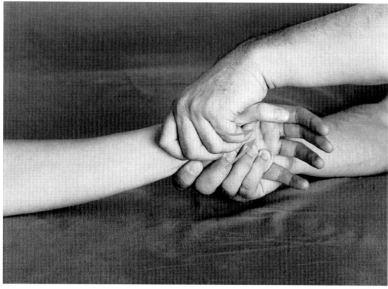

Figure 4.86   Treatment of the flexor retinaculum (from the palmar direction).

possible. The effect on the nerve's sheath can be increased by pressure against the elbow joint and by changing the angle at which the patient's forearm is flexed. In this manner, we achieve a direct stretching of the fascia of the pronator quadratus.

Step 5: Treatment of the flexor retinaculum

Patient   Supine, both legs extended.

Therapist   Standing to the side at the level of the patient's hips.

Contact   Both hands surround the carpals to be treated.

Action   The therapist's thumb presses against the head of the ulna and the end of the radius as if to slide both longitudinal bones away from the carpals. At the same time, both of the therapist's index and middle fingers strongly compress the patient's carpal tunnel and exercise a drastic stretching force on the layers of the palm. In this manner, we have the opportunity to affect different

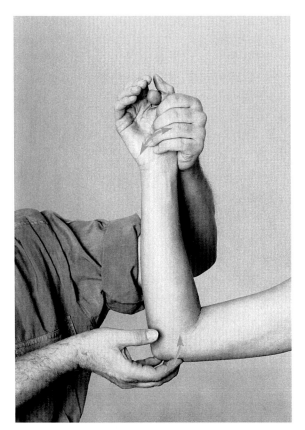

Figure 4.87 Direct influence on the median nerve within the carpal tunnel.

layers of tissue at the same time. Precisely stated, we are treating the interior of the carpal tunnel in an indirect manner in that we are moving the origin and insertion of the flexor retinaculum together while we subject the exterior tension layers that run over the joint and end in the palm of the hand to a direct treatment.

Step 6: Direct influence on the median nerve below the carpal tunnel

Patient Supine, both legs extended.

Therapist Standing to the side at the level of the patient's pectoral girdle.

Contact With the fingertips of one hand on the medial and lateral condyles of the elbow joint, with the ring finger of the other hand at the point at which the median nerve leaves the carpal tunnel distally.

Action It is recommended that the median nerve be treated directly at the point at which it passes the tunnel. It is best if we place the patient's elbow with the medial and lateral epicondyles vertically on our fingertips. With our right hand, we search for the point at which the median nerve leaves the carpal tunnel, produce as direct as possible a contact with the "nerve line," and modify the contact in the transverse and longitudinal direction. While modifying the quality of the touch on the median nerve, we allow gravity to lower the patient's forearm onto our supporting fingers as if we were trying to reduce the distance of the nerve line between the carpal tunnel and the elbow joint. The contact on the elbow then acts like a mini-trampoline in the interior of the joint, while an alternating tensional force is exerted on the nerve on the other side of the carpal tunnel. With some skill we will thus be able to guide the nerve into a subtle sliding motion within its fascial environment.

> In order to have reliable results from such treatments, it is helpful to become acquainted with the anatomical variations of the median nerve (e.g. Lanz 1987).

Additional remarks

The goal of a manual treatment of carpal tunnel syndrome is to achieve a positive change in the pressure gradient between the nerve and its adjacent boundary layers. This treatment is directed exclusively at a pattern of symptoms that arises from overloading. The treatment steps described concentrate on the fascial tissue bed of the median nerve as it runs between the shoulder region and the hand. The prognosis for a successful treatment is good as long as the compression in the tunnel primarily affects the sensory fibers, i.e. the fibers that spatially constitute the largest portion of the median nerve. As soon as motor functions are affected, the danger of lasting damage is present.

Carpal tunnel syndrome caused by a mechanical-traumatic effect should be referred to a surgeon immediately. This is particularly true in cases in which damage to the ulnar nerve in Guyon's canal is present as well.

In any event, neurological examination to accompany treatment is advisable in order to guarantee objective information regarding progress of treatment.

4.5   LOWER EXTREMITY: THIGH, LOWER LEG, AND FOOT

Aspects of form

Upon closer observation of the fascial and membrane system, chronic structural problems of an organism should not only be classified as local restrictions of movement and changes to tissue; rather, they should also be classified into the overarching structural patterns of muscular coordination and comprehensive tone patterns of the connective tissue. For this reason, in the case of chronic problems, it is not sufficient to treat the local complex of symptoms. For some acute problems, the precise treatment of a few individual elements is sometimes sufficient. However, in the case of chronic problems that have existed over a period of time, the circumstances are different. However once the compensations for local dysfunctions have exceeded a critical threshold, they develop their own problem dynamic, which continues to exist even if the original problem has been successfully treated. We try to be as precise as possible with detailed corrections within the problem zone but combine this with a global correction of the cohesive form of the body's structure.

This cohesion may be studied by way of example on the lower extremity with pelvic and back structures. An onset of arthrosis in the hip joint will influence the movement pattern in the lower leg and, over the long term, change the fascial, membrane and band structures of the ankle joint. Damage to the knee joint will not only impact the joint's function, but will cause a change in coordination over entire sections of the body. If they exist long enough, changes of this type will produce new tone patterns of the musculature and finally influence the fasciae as well.

One characteristic of the connective tissue system is that, as a three-dimensional network, it allows for compensatory changes in all spatial directions. So, the altered tone pattern of one leg

can affect the pelvis and thus involve the back as well. However, this process can occur in reverse as well: a structural weakness in the back forces one leg or both legs into a compensatory movement pattern and thus causes a long-term change to the fascial network.

Thus, there is an interdependency between the local hypotonic or hypertonic tension patterns of a problem zone and a larger context of form. For the lower extremity, this context is primarily relevant in standing and walking.

From an anatomical perspective, the close connection between the myofascial complex of the upper leg and pelvis is responsible for this fact. On the posterior side of the thigh, there is a direct connection between the fascia of the leg and the ligaments of the pelvis: at the ramus of the ischium, the fasciae of the biceps femoris muscle and the adductors unite with the strong cords of the sacrotuberous ligament. The layers coming from the distal side act on the lower edge of the pelvis with a massive longitudinal pull. In this manner, the tension pattern of the posterior side of the thigh becomes the determining factor in the tilting of the pelvis around the hip axis.

Once additional increased tension initiates from the adductor group, the ischial bones are no longer able to move apart from one another during sitting, and the pelvis retains a posterior tilt during the most various sequences of movement. The "posterior tilt" becomes the determining posture pattern.[6]

As a result, the curvature of the lumbar spine is reduced. Seen from the side, a flat back results while, on the level of the vertebral bodies, a direct curve occurs between the last lumbar vertebra and the upper edge of the sacrum instead of the curvature. As soon as a lasting structural image of the structure of the body has resulted from this, the organ column of the pelvic and abdominal cavities will respond as well:

● In men, the posterior tilt of the pelvis and the reduction of the distance between the ischial rami increases the pressure on the prostate because more of the weight of the

[6]See the detailed description in Flury and Harder (1988).

Figure 4.88 Median section of the pelvis.

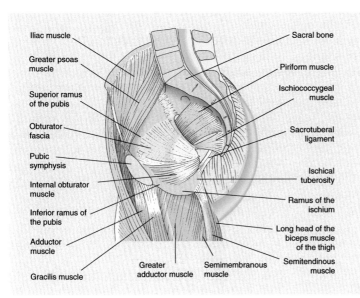

Iliac muscle

Greater psoas
muscle

Superior ramus
of the pubis

Obturator
fascia

Pubic
symphysis

Internal obturator
muscle

Inferior ramus of
the pubis

Adductor
muscle

Gracilis muscle

Greater
adductor muscle

Semimembranous
muscle

Sacral bone

Piriform muscle

Ischiococcygeal
muscle

Sacrotuberal
ligament

Ischical
tuberosity

Ramus of the
ischium

Long head of the
biceps muscle
of the thigh

Semitendinous
muscle

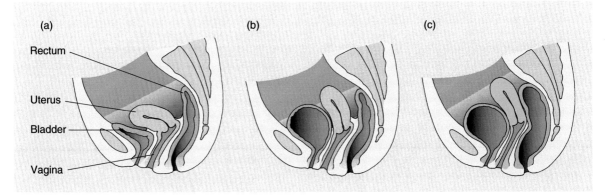

(a)   (b)   (c)

Rectum

Uterus

Bladder

Vagina

Figure 4.89 Competition for space between the uterus, rectum, and bladder: (a) with an empty bladder and empty rectum; (b) with a full bladder and empty rectum; and (c) with a full bladder and full rectum.

intraperitoneal organs is placed on it and the pubic bone pushes the bladder somewhat farther backwards over the prostate.

- In women, the uterus tends toward a posterior tilt while a part of the small intestine appears to push upward over the pubic bone and the intraperitoneal space expands backwards onto the retroperitoneal end section of the bowel. It is possible that altered tensile forces of the uterovaginal septum acting on the cervix are responsible for the tendency toward posterior displacement of the uterus. It is possible that a reduction of the retrouterine area, the so-called

Douglas space, develops and a pressure effect shows up on the sections of the large intestine located behind the uterus.

We have already been able to see that the tension relationships at the lower edge of the pelvis are responsible for tilting around the hip axis (see section 4.1) and that the posterior tilt is associated with a reduction in lumbar lordosis (see section 4.6). As a rule, this reduction is not without consequences for the sections of the back and spine located above it. Changes to one curved section of the spine bring changes to all of the other sections as well. By the sinking of the lower pelvic organs, a tensile effect on the front of the spine occurs that must be caught by the autonomic musculature with increased tone. This causes forced tensions and compressions in the intervertebral region to occur simultaneously.

Because of these circumstances and interdependencies, it can be seen that, for example, the roots of an acute, recurring ischialgia may well be found in the tension patterns of the lower extremities. For this reason, the treatment techniques described in this chapter are not only extremity techniques, but belong to the armory of pelvic and back techniques as well.

Anatomy of the fascia of the thigh

In anatomical literature, reference is repeatedly made to the fact that only a portion of the mobility that is typical for the upper extremity is available to the lower extremity. Compared with the dynamic arm, which is dominated by the grasping function, the leg has a clearly pronounced static component. This fact is revealed in the determining fascia of the thigh, the fascia lata. In some sections, it shows a mesh-like density of tissue that is not found in the region of the upper extremity even in the presence of the greatest pressure. The greatest density of the intersecting fibers of the fascia lata is found in the lateral section of the upper leg. This is because the fascia has a unique function to perform here: its increased basic tension catches the immense pressure acting on the thigh during standing and walking. By its existence, the fascia lata prevents the femur from flexing outward. Functionally, it works like an interosseus membrane that has been displaced toward the outside. The density of collagen fibers in the fascia lata is so strongly pronounced on the side of the leg that, at first glance, one tends to doubt the efficacy of manually influencing such tough layers. However, upon closer examination, we recognize that the deep layer of the fascia lata has a high degree of elasticity and movability that allows manual influence to appear quite plausible.

The fascia lata surrounds the entire thigh. In its upper part, where it is connected to the inguinal ligament and iliac crest, it is a component of the gluteal fascia and thus part of the connective tissue bridge between the lower extremity and the pelvis. With its distal branches, it connects to the superficial fascia of the knee and the periosteum of

the tibia and influences knee joint function there because individual fibers are connected to the capsule.

As has been mentioned above, the fascia lata has a considerable tissue density in its lateral portion, known as the iliotibial tract, and thus has the appearance of a flat aponeurosis. To a certain degree we find this tissue density in the dorsal region as well, although without the aponeurotic structure. In contrast, in the ventral and medial region of the upper leg, the fascia lata is very thin. On the medial side, it manifests as part of the fascial covering of the adductor group. It is therefore part of a fascial group that acts as a displacement layer during muscular activity.

Although the fibers of the fascia lata have a ring-shaped orientation, they cover only part of the thigh. Predominately, they connect to the intermuscular septa and are thus anchored in the deep layers of the leg. However, there is also a smaller portion of the fibers with a low level of tensile strength that encircles the entire thigh. These fibers are located directly below the subcutaneous layer.

The core layer of the fascia lata is so tough that it can inhibit the mobility of the muscle fibers. The change in the muscles' shape in flexion and extension is only possible because another loose sliding layer is located between the actual fascial layer and the musculature. We find a comparable sliding layer in the front and rear region of the thigh between the subcutis and the fascia. In this manner, the solid, difficult-to-stretch elements of the fascia lata are embedded on the surface and in the deep layers of the thigh in sliding layers with a greater elasticity. I think that this results in a kind of "combinational elasticity" for these fascial layers, which at first glance appear to be impossible to stretch.

It is important for treatment techniques that we keep in mind that the fascia lata does not function only as a superficial layer. In the deep layers, it is linked to the intermuscular septa of the thigh.

Moreover, there are a few other peculiarities in the region of the fascia lata that are worthy of attention for treatment practice: the muscles embedded in the fascia lata have their own directional fascial sheaths, inside of which the muscles can slide somewhat with the aid of an epimysium. In isolated

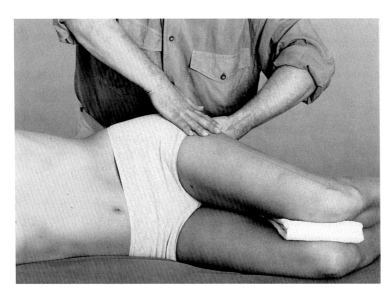

Figure 4.90   Treatment of the fascia lata (lateral layer).

cases, this epimysium is a cylindrical fascial tube, such as in the case of the sartorius muscle. This is a special form that is typical of diagonal muscle paths. Also, the fascia of the sternocleidomastoid muscle has a similar position in the region of the fasciae of the neck. We find a comparable invagination in the case of the gracilis muscle. Finally, there is one other peculiarity of the fasciae of the lower extremity that has significance for the circulatory system. Von Lanz and Wachsmuth (1972: 48) have shown that the large vascular routes of the leg are located not inside the musculature, but rather between the "stiff-walled fascial tubes."

The musculature requires the resistance of the stiff fascial tubes in order to produce their characteristic effect as muscular pumps on the accompanying veins of the arteries.

Treatment techniques

Treatment of the fascia lata (lateral layer)

Patient   Lying on one side with knees flexed, small pillow between the knees.

Therapist   Standing next to the patient's hips.

Contact   With a slightly closed fist at the medial end of the subgluteal, horizontal part of the fascia lata (see Figure 4.94), with the other hand right on the posterior edge of the longitudinal path of the iliotibial tract.

Action   With an elastically closed fist, we gently push through the skin and fatty layers just under the gluteal fold in order to produce a flat hand contact on the seat halter of the fascia lata. We maintain a flat contact at this point without sliding. The holding surface that results is significant because the seat halter has a unique, three-dimensional branching, specifically outward in the direction of the skin, laterally toward the iliotibial tract, and medially until the tuberosity of the ischium. Thus, it connects the subcutaneous layer, the aponeurosis, and the periosteum. With the palm of the other hand, we press on the posterior edge of the longitudinal path of the iliotibial tract, first anteriorly in a diagonal direction. The pressure that we exert goes barely past the outer edge of the femur. We follow the tract along its entire length with strong contact up to the layer of the head of the fibula. It is important to adapt the contact to the density of the fibers and the sliding layer located below them in order to prevent a squeezing effect on the bones.

Treatment of the fascia lata (posterior layer) and the fasciae of the biceps femoris, semimembranosus, and semitendinosus muscles

Patient   Supine, one leg flexed, one knee pulled up and held with both hands.

Therapist   Standing at the level of the diaphragm, facing distally.

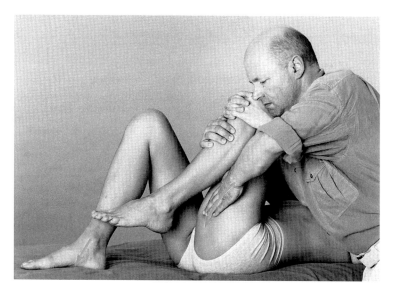

Figure 4.91   Treatment of the fascia lata (posterior layer) and the fasciae of the biceps femoris, semimembranosus, and semitendinosus muscles, first treatment step.

Contact   Using the shoulder to provide counter-pressure on the patient's pulled-up knee, strong, sliding contact in the posterior layers of the fascia.

Action   We ask the patient to hold the knee with both hands so that the thigh rotates minimally inward. It is important for the other leg to maintain a good functional contact with the treatment table so that the orientation of the hip axis remains horizontal, even if massive pressure is exerted on the posterior side of the thigh. The therapist's shoulder now leans against the patient's pulled-up knee so as to apply some of the therapist's weight against this knee. At the same time, the majority of the weight of the therapist's upper body is transferred into the palms, and the therapist exerts a slow stretching force on the posterior layer of the fascia lata. This stretching motion extends over the entire posterior side of the thigh, beginning just below the hollow of the knee and ending at the point where the gluteal fascia overlaps the biceps femoris.

In a second treatment step, we produce contact specifically between the posterior boundary of the iliotibial tract and the biceps femoris by reaching with our second hand between the biceps femoris and semitendinosus muscles. We exert strong, slowly gliding pressure, which this time acts deeply into the grooves between the muscles. This contact is less two-dimensional than in the first step. In the case of a high degree of muscle tone, it is advisable to use the edge of the hand.

This technique can be applied analogously to the semitendinosus and semimembranosus, while we work between the semimembranosus and adductor magnus muscles.

> The efficacy of this technique depends on the careful graduation of the very strong pressure as well as the coordination of this pressure with the pull that the patient is exerting on the upper leg. The pull should be just strong enough that the ischial bones expand somewhat, but the hip joint should not be compressed too strongly.

Treatment of the deep layer of the iliotibial tract in connection with the subgluteal, horizontal part of the fascia lata

Patient   Supine, one leg pulled up with both hands.

Therapist   Standing distally of the hip axis, facing in the cranial direction.

Contact   One palm on the upper third of the iliotibial tract with the second phalanx of the index and middle fingers of the other hand on the medial portion of the subgluteal, horizontal part of the fascia lata.

Action   The therapist's hands move in opposite directions. In order to protect the therapist's own neck, it is essential to keep the shoulders loose and

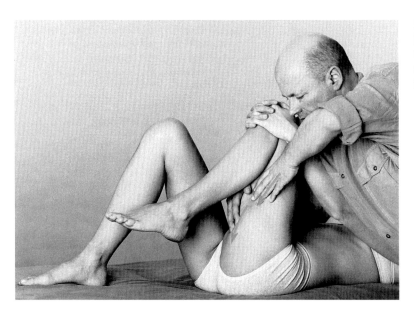

Figure 4.92   Treatment of the fascia lata (posterior layer) and the fasciae of the biceps femoris, semimembranosus, and semitendinosus muscles, second treatment step.

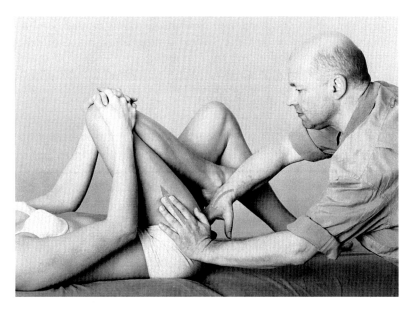

Figure 4.93   Treatment of the deep layer of the iliotibial tract in connection with the subgluteal, horizontal part of the fascia lata

for the movement impulse to originate from the elbows. The palm on the tract slides freely, with the pressure moving first through the tough superficial fascial layers into the sliding intermediate layer, and then acting almost parallel to the exterior of the femur. In no way should we attempt to pull on the exterior layers. The contact by both phalanges on the subgluteal, horizontal part of the fascia lata wanders slowly. It works in slow motion, as if we were constantly waiting for the bone to

respond to the shifting pull and pressure forces and readjust itself in its fascial bed.

Treatment of the fascia lata (medial layer) and the investing fascia of the adductors

Patient   Lying on one side, the lower leg almost extended, the upper leg to be treated slightly flexed.

Therapist   Standing behind the patient at the level of the thigh.

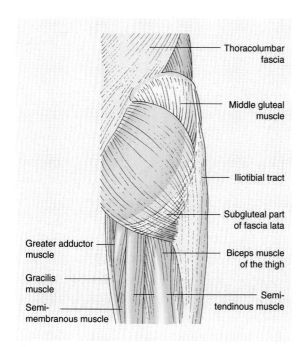

Figure 4.94   Fiber orientation of the subgluteal, horizontal part of the fascia lata.

Contact   With one hand on the medial side of the knee at the level of the insertion of the sartorius, gracilis, and the tendon of the semitendinosus; with the other hand between the fascial layers of the adductor magnus and the semimembranosus muscles.

Action   The patient's ankle is allowed to rest on the therapist's flexed thigh while the therapist surrounds the patient's knee on the medial side with one hand. With the fingertips of the other hand, the therapist now absorbs the weight of the thigh and carefully reaches through the fascia lata, which is very thin here, in order to arrive behind the sartorius muscle at the boundary of the fascial sheath of the adductor magnus and the semimembranosus muscles. No contact is established here with the blood vessels or the saphenous nerve at the level of the intermuscular septum. The therapist first waits for the tissue response and then, using the weight of the thigh, gradually reaches between the fascial tubes. At this point we maintain contact and now we modify it with our other hand by slight abduction and adduction of the angle of our contact. Subsequently, we follow the course of the muscles in a slowly gliding manner in the cranial direction as if we were trying to separate their fascial sheaths from one another. The efficacy of this technique can be increased if we ask the patient to accompany our manipulation by bending the hips, i.e. pulling the knee up slightly parallel to the treatment table and extending it again somewhat, specifically just after we have produced an strong contact between the fasciae of the adductor muscle and semitendinosus muscle. It is possible to treat the fascial boundaries between the adductor magnus and the gracilis muscle in a corresponding manner.

Because the fascia lata is usually only very thinly pronounced on the inside of the leg, we should ensure that the stretching effect reaches through the superficial layer into the deep layer without overstretching the superficial layer. Over the gracilis muscle and adductor magnus, the group fascia of the adductors functions simultaneously as a superficial fascia. For this reason, it is helpful to use the weight of the leg to be treated for the purpose of accessing deeper layers. In the manner, we are able to protect the nerves running parallel to the sartorius muscle in spite of the strong contact.

Treatment of the anterior layer of the fascia lata in combination with the posterior layer

Patient   Supine, one leg flexed, the other leg extended.

Therapist   Sitting at the level of the patient's hips, facing distally.

Contact   With one palm on the front of the thigh and with the fingertips of the other hand lateral of the group fascia of the adductors.

Action   First, we produce a flat contact with the fascia on the front of the leg, which is relatively thin there. As the same time, our fingertips reach into the tissue behind the leg, lateral to the adductor fascia and toward the femur. While we now cross the fascial fibers with flat contact in the distal direction on the front of the leg, the far more

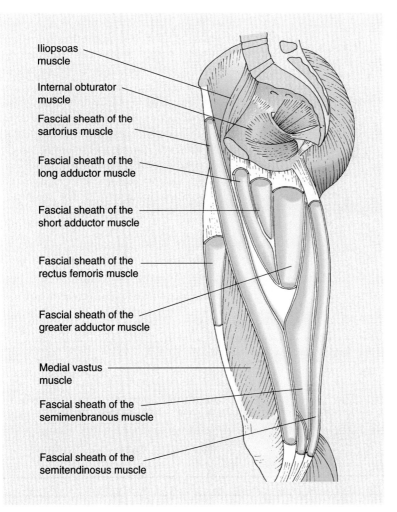

Iliopsoas muscle

Internal obturator muscle

Fascial sheath of the sartorius muscle

Fascial sheath of the long adductor muscle

Fascial sheath of the short adductor muscle

Fascial sheath of the rectus femoris muscle

Fascial sheath of the greater adductor muscle

Medial vastus muscle

Fascial sheath of the semimenbranous muscle

Fascial sheath of the semitendinosus muscle

Figure 4.95 Fascial tubes of the thigh from the medial direction (according to Benninghoff).

specific contact on the rear side wanders in the cranial direction as if we were trying to produce a groove between the adductors and the semitendinosus muscle. As we do so, we ask the patient to alternately flex and extend the knee slightly. On the front, the contact remains gently sliding, while we use the weight of the leg on the rear side, which has more strongly pronounced fasciae, to slide more strongly and very slowly.

Although we are working on the front and rear of the leg with different qualities of touch, we have a common technical strategy. In both regions, we are "waiting" for the response of the tissue and the bone connected to the fascia lata by way of the intermuscular septa before we intensify the contact. By doing so, we are respecting a fundamental rule of fascial and membrane techniques, which states that we should give an impulse into the superficial layers only strongly enough that the deeper layers can follow the response of the superficial layers.

Anatomy of the fasciae of the lower leg and foot

Analogously to the upper extremity, we find a superficial fascia that is connected to the deep layers in the calf as well. There is a direct connection

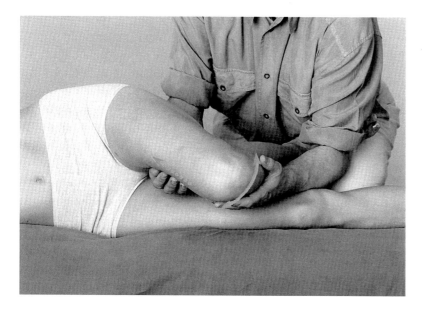

Figure 4.96   Treatment of the fascia lata (medial layer) and the investing fascia of the adductors.

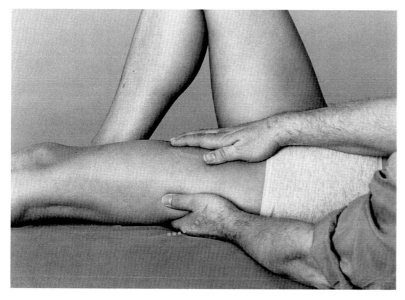

Figure 4.97   Treatment of the anterior layer of the fascia lata in combination with the posterior layer.

between the superficial and deep crural fascia in that one anterior and one posterior intermuscular septum runs inward from the superficial layer. Similarly to the forearm, longitudinal displacement of the bones is prevented in the lower leg by a strong interosseus membrane. Along with the tibia and fibula, this membrane separates the extensor musculature located in the front section of the lower leg from the flexor musculature located in the rear section of the lower leg. In addition to this osteofibrous separation, a fibrous chamber for

the triceps surae of the calf is also formed by the deep lamina of the crural fascia, forming an additional chamber between the superficial and deep plantar flexors.

A few peculiarities of the crural fascia are of importance for the techniques described below. From a purely mechanical viewpoint, its superficial layer is closely connected to the periosteum of the tibia. A connection to the fibula by way of the front intermuscular septum is present as well. From a neurological viewpoint, since Staubesand's

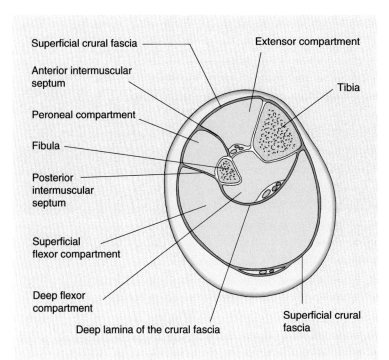

Superficial crural fascia

Anterior intermuscular
septum

Peroneal compartment

Fibula

Posterior
intermuscular
septum

Superficial
flexor compartment

Deep flexor
compartment

Deep lamina of the crural fascia

Extensor compartment

Tibia

Superficial crural
fascia

Figure 4.98   Fascial and muscular canals
of the lower leg in cross-section at the
level of the lower third.

research, the fascia has prompted far-reaching consideration (Staubesand and Li 1996; Schleip 2003): Staubesand found contractile fibers in the crural fascia. Using altered tensile stress, the fascia could therefore modify the tough spatial delimiters in the lower leg down into the interconnection of membranes and periostea.

This sort of modification would have a substantial influence on the muscle tone because the fascia serves as the origin of the muscle in the proximal direction.

For treatment techniques, it is helpful to pay attention to the different formations of the fascia. Depending on the level of load, the fascia on the superficial and deep levels will develop in a more or less fibrous fashion. It can sometimes be so stiff that it can hardly be distinguished from the adjacent musculature. In individual deep sections, it can also function as a simple displacement layer. Von Lanz and Wachsmuth (1972: 303) have referred to the fact that the deep crural fascia doubles over the tuberosity of calcaneus while farther in the cranial direction it becomes quite delicate and, in the proximal direction, it frequently becomes a simple "displacement device."

This dissimilarity in the morphology of the fascia requires an extremely precise differentiation in the quality of touch when treating the lower leg.

There is one other characteristic of the crural fascia that requires a particular treatment technique. At its lower end, where it comprises only a relatively thin layer, it transitions seamlessly into the retinacula; it forms regular guiding canals into which the tendon sheaths are embedded, in the front it forms them for the extensor tendons along with two retinacula and in the rear it forms them for the flexor tendons.

Each of the retinacula continues on the rear of the foot and the sole of the foot into the fascial layers of the foot. Thus, the retinacula provide a connection to the plantar aponeurosis in the distal direction and to the crural fascia in the proximal direction. For the treatment of these structures, it is important to bear in mind that the retinacula do not represent a separate band structure; rather, they are a functionally determined local thickening of fascia. Correspondingly, any effect on their tough fibrous structure is always also an effect of the overall fascial complex of the leg and foot.

In contrast to the retinacula, the fascia on the rear of the foot is thin and easily displaceable. This layer should be included in treatment only in the case of an extremely high arch of the foot and, even in these cases, treatment should occur on the adjacent retinacula to the greatest extent possible so as to protect the tendon sheaths located farther in the distal direction on the back of the foot. Caution is advised on the sole of the foot as well for the plantar fascia, which usually has a strong structure. Only in the case of extremely high arches of the foot should we attempt to have a massive effect on the plantar fascia. Because the foot has lost its grasping function over the course of human development and muscles have been converted into ligaments, its form and structure are determined substantially more by bands than by fasciae.

Treatment techniques for the axes of hinge joints at the level of the ankle, knee, and hip joints

The following techniques can be traced back to Ida Rolf. These techniques have proven themselves primarily in the treatment of decreased flexion or extension function in joints of the lower extremity. I have achieved the best results in treatment after surgical interventions and after immobilization (splint or cast). In my opinion, the efficacy of these techniques is due to the successful combination of a direct effect on the connective tissue and precisely coordinated active movement on the part of the patient. These methods are based on the notion that, in the vicinity of a joint, we will only ever be able to reach some of the tissue layers using direct contact. Another part of those layers can be accessed only in an indirect manner using active movement by the patient.

These techniques can be varied in a variety of ways. However, they always follow a clear treatment strategy: the therapist's hands create several fixed points, or more accurately fixed surfaces of the deep fascia, and exercise pressure in such a way that the joint positions itself as normally as possible. In other words, the therapist holds the joint in the normal hinge axis position to the greatest extent possible. Then the therapist asks the patient to slowly perform flexion and extension movements of the affected joint while the therapist

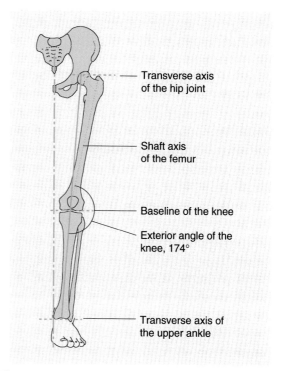

Figure 4.99   Hinge joint axes of the ankle, knee, and hip joints.

continues to hold the joint within the hinge axis in a very decisive manner. This causes an activation of muscle fibers that are usually involved in movement only to a limited extent as well as an orientation of the fasciae and membranes that also corresponds to the hinge joint axis.

Treatment of the ankle and knee joint using the hinge joint axis technique in three steps

First step

Patient   Supine, one leg flexed, one leg extended in such a way that the heel extends over the edge of the treatment table.

Therapist   Sitting at the foot, facing in the cranial direction.

Contact   With the surface of the distal phalanges of both hands at the point at which the inferior extensor retinaculum intersects with the tendon sheaths, while both thumbs support the arch of the foot just in front of the heel.

Action   The therapist uses the distal phalanges to reach in a two-dimensional manner toward the inferior extensor retinacula of the lower legs and, at the same time, supports both longitudinal arches from below with the thumbs. The therapist asks the patient to adduct first the toes and then the foot. Subsequently, first the foot should be stretched and then the toes. During this entire sequence of movements, the therapist maintains strong contact with the retinacula and fixes the hinge joint axis. While the patient repeats the sequence of movements several times, the therapist stretches the fibers.

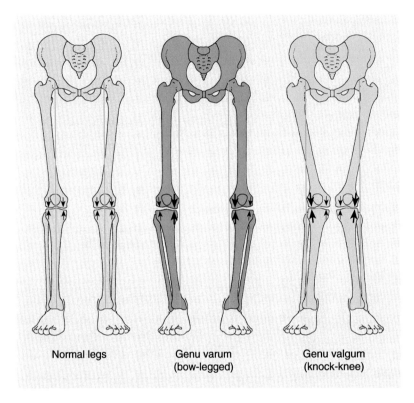

Normal legs   Genu varum (bow-legged)   Genu valgum (knock-knee)

Figure 4.100 Load on the knee joint with a normal hinge axis and an altered hinge axis.

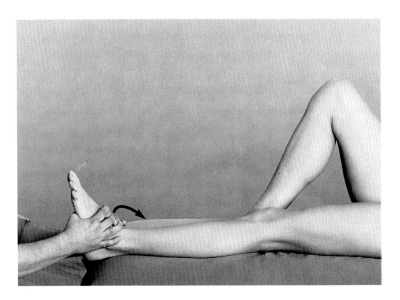

Figure 4.101 Treatment of the ankle and knee joint using the hinge joint axis technique, first treatment step.

Second step

In a continuing treatment step, the therapist uses the ulna, just below the elbow joint, to contact the medial side of the retinaculum, while strongly surrounding the lateral side of the ankle. At the same time, the therapist's sternum supports the foot as if the sole of the patient's foot were trying

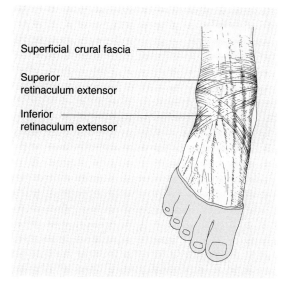

Superficial crural fascia

Superior retinaculum extensor

Inferior retinaculum extensor

Figure 4.102   Fiber orientation of the retinacula at the transition between the lower leg and foot.

to push against the therapist's thoracic cavity. The therapist asks the patient to move the knee approximately 5 cm toward the ceiling and, at the same time, moves the patient's foot upward using the sternum so that a correct hinge joint movement occurs at the same time in the ankle, knee, and hip joints. The therapist remains in extremely energetic contact so that the hinge joint axis remains precisely in the same position as soon as the patient raises and then lowers the knee. More simply, the therapist exerts pressure inward using the ulna and the hand, compressing the joint while maintaining the hinge joint axis while the patient provides a correcting impulse with the movement described above. Depending on the extent of the deviation from the hinge joint, this sequence of movements may have to be repeated up to five times. The efficacy of this method can be increased by asking the patient to perform the movement only in a minimal fashion and finally, following an idea by Moshe Feldenkrais, advising the patient to only imagine performing the movement.

Third step

Patient   Same position as above.

Therapist   Standing, one knee flexed on the treatment table.

Figure 4.103   Treatment of the ankle and knee joint using the hinge joint axis technique, second treatment step.

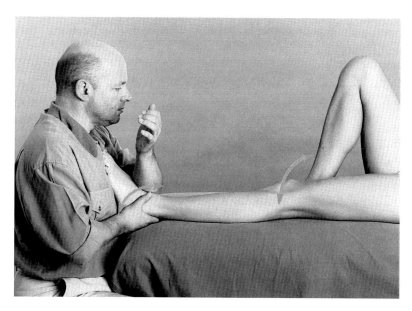

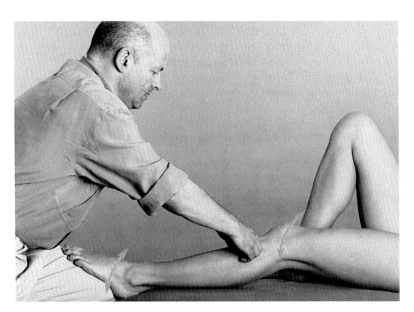

Figure 4.104 Treatment of the ankle and knee joint using the hinge joint axis technique, third treatment step.

Contact With the therapist's knee at the sole of the patient's foot, with the second phalanges of the index and middle fingers of both hands below the hinge joint of the knee.

Action While the therapist's knee is pressed against the sole of the patient's foot, the second phalanges of the index and middle fingers of both hands are used to contact below the client's knee, specifically medially at the level of the patellar tendon and laterally on the level of the cranial portion of the tibialis anterior. On the medial side, the fascial fibers are diagonally oriented between the front edge of the tibia and the interior of the knee; on the lateral side, they are oriented almost vertically to the head of the fibula. The therapist initially maintains the contact while the patient raises the knee against the therapist's pressure. The contact on the sole of the foot is maintained so that a guidance of the joint occurs in a hinging motion. While the patient repeats this sequence of movements several times, the therapist begins slowly to intersect the fascial fibers below the knee at both contact points: horizontally on the lateral side and in a crescent-shaped line against the diagonal path of the fascia on the medial side (see Figure 4.104). Even during this strong contact with the fascia, the guidance of the hinge joints at the ankle and knee must be maintained.

The efficacy of the hinge joint technique depends on the precision of the guided movements. It is important to position the leg as if standing with the heel on the floor so that the three hinge planes at the ankle, knee, and hip run parallel to one another. This is only possible to a certain extent in the case of pronounced knock-knee or bow legs. In cases of drastic deviation from the hinge joint, we leave the leg in its deviation and ask the patient to perform the movement for only a few millimeters.

The three treatment steps described above can be varied by selecting the lateral and medial contact points above one hinge joint and below the next highest hinge joint.

Treatment of the superficial layer of the crural fascia

Patient Lying supine, one leg flexed.

Therapist Sitting at the foot.

Contact The therapist's shoulder supports the sole of the foot. With one hand, the therapist slightly

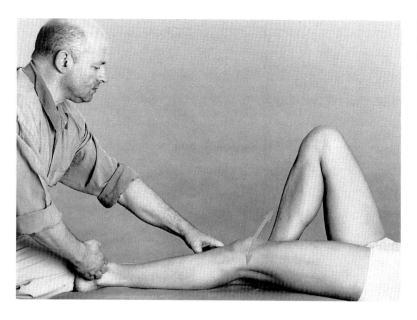

Figure 4.105   Treatment of the ankle and knee joint using the hinge joint axis technique (variations).

lifts the lower leg by grasping the crural fascia in the distal direction from the medial portion of the gastrocnemius muscle and the fingertips (medial side) and the thumb (lateral side) of the other hand surround the head of the fibula.

Action   The foot of the patient's slightly raised leg is in contact with the therapist's shoulder. The therapist surrounds the head of the fibula while using the other hand to produce a flat contact on the rear side of the lower leg. The therapist uses the shoulder contact to move the patient's ankle passively while using the contact with both hands to move the knee and hip joints in the movement direction of the hinge joint axis. While doing so, the therapist follows the deviations from the hinge joint axis passively, with "listening" and without reducing contact with the fascia.

In the case of genu valgum, the leg will move farther into the knock-knee configuration. The therapist follows the movement until it has almost come to a stop and, at this moment, applies a sustained impulse into the fascial tissue and/or the connecting ligaments at the head of the fibula in order to then follow the leg in its countermovement.

In the case of genu varum, the leg usually moves somewhat more strongly into the bow-legged shape. In this case, it is better to maintain contact

on the medial side of the tibia instead of on the head of the fibula and to follow the leg farther into the genu varum.

In both cases, genu valgum and genu varum, the indirect guidance into joint fixation should be combined with the direct impulse applied to the fascia. The effect presumably arises because we are simultaneously exerting influence on the ligaments near the joint and the insertion of the crural fascia in the proximal position of the tibia and fibula.

Treatment of the interosseous membrane of the lower leg

Patient   Supine, both legs extended.

Therapist   Sitting at the feet.

Contact   Initially, with two fingertips of one hand from behind on the farthest distal point of the lateral malleolus, with the fingertips of the other hand also from behind, slightly above the distal fifth of the tibia.

Action   The therapist's fingertips gently push the lateral malleolus from the distal and posterior directions precisely parallel to the fiber orientation of the anterior tibiofibular ligament so that the lateral malleolus slightly approaches the lower

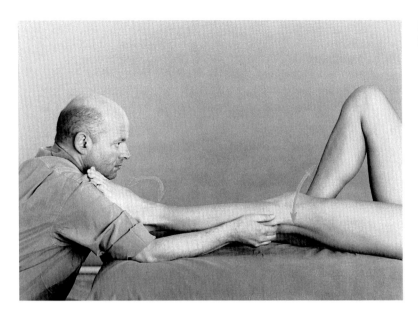

Figure 4.106 Treatment of the superficial layer of the crural fascia.

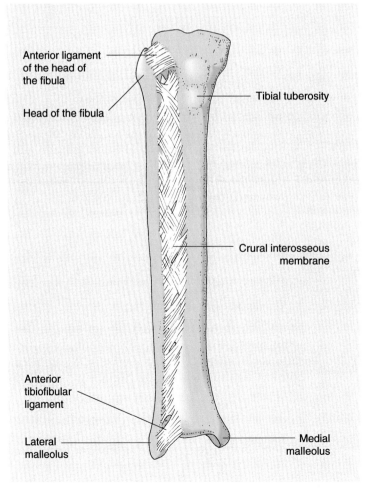

Figure 4.107 Interosseus membrane of the lower leg from the anterior direction.

Anterior ligament of the head of the fibula

Head of the fibula

Tibial tuberosity

Crural interosseous membrane

Anterior tibiofibular ligament

Lateral malleolus

Medial malleolus

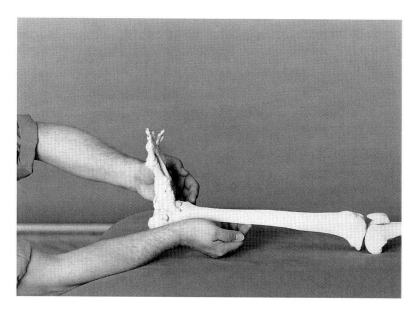

Figure 4.108   Treatment of the interosseous membrane of the lower leg.

medial end of the tibia and the band running between them relaxes somewhat. During this, the fingers of the therapist's second hand surround the inner edge of the tibia from behind and guide the entire bone gently toward the contact point of the other hand. While this causes the tibia to be very slightly displaced in the distal direction, the fibula will go into either rotation or a longitudinal shift depending on the dominant fiber tension of the interosseus membrane. The therapist follows this movement, which occurs spatially in several steps, while the quality of contact achieves in the patient as deep as possible a relaxation and reduction in tone of the exterior muscle layers. The therapist accepts the weight of the lower leg more and more and, while doing so, performs the "listening" described above until the movement comes to a stop.

This technique can be varied by using mobility tests to find the point with the strongest restriction between the two bones of the lower leg. We frequently find this point in the region of an old fracture. In practice, it is important to ensure that the contact points that we select with both hands are diagonal to one another so that both of our hands can follow the dominant direction of pull and, in so doing, be able to align them relative to one another in their muscular and fascial beds. This technique can be applied accordingly on the upper end of the lower leg; here, we must bear in mind the almost horizontal orientation of the fibers of the anterior ligament of the head of the fibula and should therefore guide the head of the fibula almost parallel to the hinge joint of the tibia while supporting the tibia from behind.

Critical readers may doubt that this technique even affects the interosseous membrane. It is certainly correct to assume that the effect is transmitted to the deep crural fascia, which is more elastic, to its insertion in the distal portion of the bones of the lower leg, and to the corresponding muscular insertions. The following technique attempts to take this possible connection into account.

Treatment of the deep crural fascia in the overarching fascial context

Patient   Supine, both legs extended.

Therapist   Sitting at the feet.

Contact   With the side of the flexed index finger facing the thumb on the rear of the lower leg near the talus and slightly below the gastrocnemius muscle.

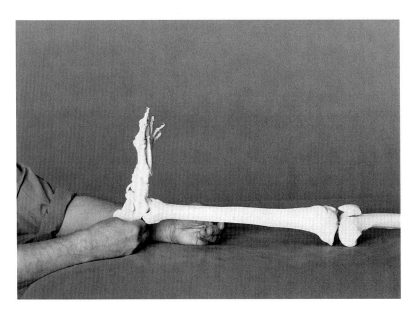

Figure 4.109   Treatment of the deep crural fascia.

Action   Both of the therapist's hands are placed on the treatment table with the outer edge and the fingers are slightly flexed. The hand applied below in the region of the talus is somewhat flatter under the patient's lower leg than the second hand so that the patient's knee is slightly raised. The therapist now gradually modifies the quality of the touch—it becomes gradually more elastic until the tone of the superficial muscles relaxes more and more and a contact is produced with the deep crural fascia. At this moment, the therapist applies a slight impulse upward, in the direction of the ceiling, as if to gently reach upward with the fingertips through the deep crural fascia. In so doing, the therapist follows any tensile forces that may occur that guide both hands together or apart while remaining constantly in strong yet elastic contact. It is as if the therapist were touching a stretched trampoline from below, tracing the tension patterns that manifest there, and noting the tensional forces working on this trampoline in order to set them against one another and gradually neutralize them. Successful neutralization can be recognized by the patient's lower leg finally resting on the therapist's fingertips in a completely motionless fashion. At this moment, it is worthwhile to gently push both contact points in the cranial direction until the resistance of the knee joint is felt. If the resistance has the same quality in the medial and lateral directions, it is advisable to remove the shear

force and break off the process. However, if we can feel a difference, we first follow the more elastic side as far as we can and wait for the reverse impulse to exert a subtle shear pulse on the side that was originally more strongly "blocked" until the lateral and medial edges of the knee offer the same amount of resistance. This is the moment of equilibrium in which we remove our touch.

TREATMENT OF THE HIP JOINT IN THE CASE OF ONSET OF ARTHROSIS

In recent years, considerable advances have been made in the implantation of artificial hip joints. The implants themselves as well as the surgical procedures have improved substantially so that today a positive long-term prognosis can be given in most cases.

The manual techniques described below are directed at two goals:

- On the one hand, the attempt should be made to optimize the transmission of pressure forces onto the hip joint, to facilitate a better distribution of joint fluid and thus slow the course of progressive changes to cartilage. In the most favorable case, it should be possible to postpone the time at which an implant is required.

- On the other hand, the treatment of the involved connective tissue structures should achieve a type of rehabilitation before the surgical intervention.

In the course of progressive arthrosis of the hip joint, considerable compensatory changes occur not only in the pelvic region, but also in the distal direction from the hip joint, primarily in the ankles. In the superior direction from the hip joint, primarily in the region of the pectoral girdle, compensatory changes to muscle tone and fascial tension may be frequently observed as well. In my practice, I have observed again and again that manual treatment as preparation for an implant, i.e. rehabilitation before the surgical intervention, is more important than postoperative care. This may be due to the fact that compensatory changes already emerge in the myofascial system at the beginning of arthrosis. These compensations manifest themselves progressively in the muscular units of the pelvis, primarily in the rotators, which connect the sacrum to the femur on the greater trochanter. After a longer period of time, these changes not only act on the musculature, but also extend to the fibers of the ligaments:

- the sacrotuberous ligament
- the sacrospinous ligament
- the obturator membrane.

If these changes are not treated before the surgical intervention, the implant will be included in the compensatory tension pattern that corresponds to the inflamed joint that was restricted in its movement. In the case of a strongly pronounced compensation pattern, the ability of the organism to adapt is overextended. In this case, we are confronted by a situation in which, in spite of a "new," functional hip, the dysfunction of the surrounding tissue continues to hinder coordinated overall function.

It is not simple to differentiate to what extent the changes mentioned above actually correspond to a compensatory pattern and to what extent they already had an effect before the onset of the arthrosis, perhaps as a mechanical component of changes to cartilage. This differentiation, however, does not play any role in our practical treatment strategy. In any event, we must treat the hip in such a way that tendencies toward "normal" pressure and tension conditions are already manifest in the myofascial units that intersect the joint capsule or have their course in its vicinity before the implantation of the artificial hip joint. In order to achieve an effective treatment result, it is necessary to combine globally applied techniques that act on the fascial complex above and below the joint capsule with techniques that influence structures inside the capsule.

Anatomy of the fasciae and membranes in the region of the hip joint

Because the hip joint is located directly at the transition between the lower extremity and the interior of the pelvis, very different myofascial units of the body components mentioned above—pelvis, legs, feet—can have an influence on the function of this joint. The joint must be able to withstand compressional forces originating from the torso as well as strong tensional forces from the lower extremity.

In the superficial layer, we encounter the anterior portion of the fascia lata. It is significant as the overarching layer for the hip joint because it is connected to the iliac crest, inguinal ligament, pubic bone, and ischial bone and continues in the distal direction to the superficial fascia of the knee (Lanz and Wachsmut 1972: 100).

In addition, the fascial sheath layers of the adductor group, which are referred to in their distal region as the pectineal fascia, are significant as the middle layer. I would speculate that these fascial sheath layers, along with the predominant tone pattern of their associated musculature, play a role in the distal portion of the hip joint. It is possible that the tensile forces that act on the medial and distal portion of the joint are responsible for the narrowing of the seam of the joint that is visible in radiographic images. It is possible that tensile forces acting in the posterior direction, i.e. the entire myofascial complex of the rotators, play a role. In the case of these layers that run posteriorly between the sacrum and the great trochanter, individual muscles have a particularly important role because they are able to intensify the compressive forces within the joint. All muscles that rotate the leg outward and that run parallel to strong ligaments should be emphasized. For example, the superior gemellus muscle, which runs from the spine of the ischium to the trochanteric fossa, should be mentioned because its fibers have an orientation that runs parallel to that of the sacrospinous ligament, which has a high tensile strength. The three-dimensional, not just two-dimensional, impact on the hip joint becomes clear when we observe that the fibers of the obturator internus muscle have an orientation parallel to that of the sacrospinous ligament. The obturator internus has a strongly pronounced fascial sheath and, in its tendinous portion, is connected to the tendons of the superior and inferior gemelli muscles where they insert into the trochanteric fossa.

In this myofascial context, the iliopsoas fascia also plays an important role. Along with the periosteum of the iliac fossa, it forms an osteofibrous tube that offers space for the iliac muscle. Von Lanz and Wachsmut (1972: 98) have pointed out that the posterior side of this tube has grown into the capsule of the hip joint.

Moreover, the interrelation of connective tissue elements of the pelvic cavity with the iliopsoas fascia is significant as well: the path of the renal fascia is in the direct vicinity of the psoas muscle. Its posterior layer is connected to the psoas fascia and the medial crus of the diaphragm (Breul 2002).

For the diagnostic evaluation of the hip joint, it is important to bear in mind that disease processes can spread by way of the renal fascia from the perirenal space in the inferior direction by way of the lacuna of muscles to the lesser trochanter. In the latter case, pain occurs in the region of the hip joint, the cause of which can be found in the perirenal space.

Finally, it should also be mentioned that the chamber of the pelvic and abdominal cavities located above the hip joint transmits pressure in the direction of the hip joint. We can only speculate as to the extent to which this transmission of pressure has unfavorable effects on the hip joint due to restrictions in organ movement. In practice, techniques that take into account the peritoneal space and the retroperitoneal concentration of connective tissue of the organs have proven useful.

In addition to the numerous layers that intersect with the hip joint outside of its capsule, the interior of the joint capsule has significance for the treatment concept described above as well. Between the head of the femur and the hip joint

capsule, there is a cushion of connective tissue and fat as well as the ligament of the head of the femur. The mobility and cushioning function of these elements play a considerable role in intracapsular distribution of fluid.

Treatment techniques

Treatment of the myofascial tension patterns that transmit onto the ischial ramus

Patient   Supine, one knee flexed.

Therapist   Sitting next to the treatment table at the level of the patient's knee.

Contact   With the flat underside of the fingertips of one hand between the origin of the adductor magnus and semitendinosus muscle as near as possible to the ischial tuberosity; at the same time, the other hand supports the entire thigh from the posterior direction.

Action   The supporting hand raises the thigh slightly so that a passive flexion of the hip and knee joint occurs. At the same time, the fingertips of the other hand gradually move between the adductor magnus and semitendinosus toward the ischial tuberosity. The passive movement of the thigh causes the contact to wander gradually inward and, once it arrives under the subgluteal, horizontal part

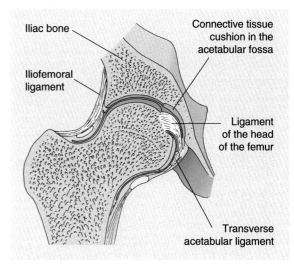

Figure 4.110   Frontal section of the right hip joint.

of the fascia lata, it should work determinedly and unyieldingly in the deep layer. As soon as the contact arrives in the deep layer between the two muscles, we can increase the efficacy by using our supporting hand to guide the entire leg passively in slight inward and outward rotations. In so doing, it is important for our contact to be applied parallel to the muscle fibers and transverse to the primary direction of the fascial fibers.

Treatment of the myofascial complex of the rotator group

Patient Supine, one leg flexed.

Therapist Sitting next to the treatment table at the level of the patient's knee.

Contact With the fingertips through the exterior gluteal muscles in the direction of the rotator

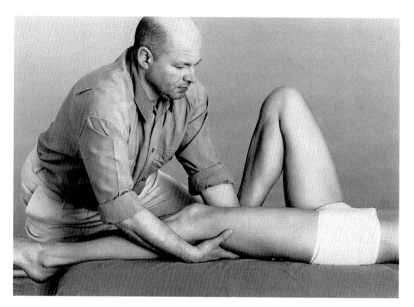

Figure **4.111** Treatment of the myofascial tension patterns that transmit onto the ischial ramus.

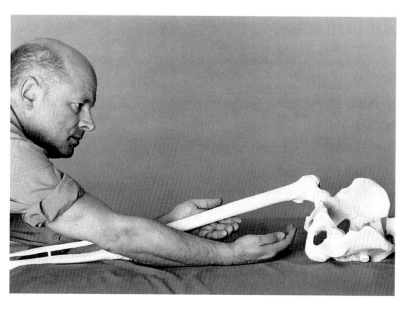

Figure **4.112** Hand position for the treatment of the right hip.

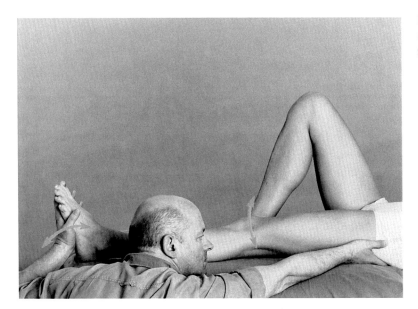

Figure 4.113   Treatment of the myofascial complex of the rotator group.

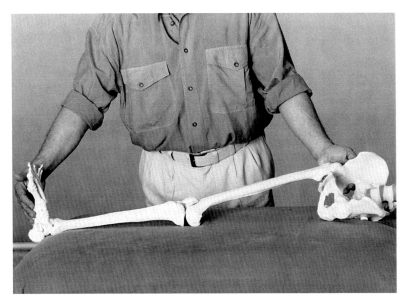

Figure 4.114   Hand position for the treatment of the right hip.

group, while the other hand maintains contact with the sole of the foot.

Action The therapist uses the patient's weight initially to reach through the superficial gluteal musculature. The contact of the therapist's fingers is placed precisely between the obturator internus and the piriformis. The pressure is thus transmitted approximately to the layers of the gemellus superior. While the other hand supports the sole of the foot in a flat manner, the patient's attention is directed toward the tactile perception of the "artificial ground" formed by our hand (this designation was originated by Moshe Feldenkrais, although he used a wood board held in both of the therapist's hands to produce the artificial floor). The patient is now asked to exert slight pressure with the soles of the feet; the therapist's hand provides counterpressure so the patient's knee is raised somewhat. During this process, the therapist

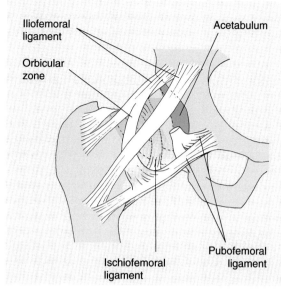

Figure 4.115 Reinforcing ligaments of the joint capsule of the hip.

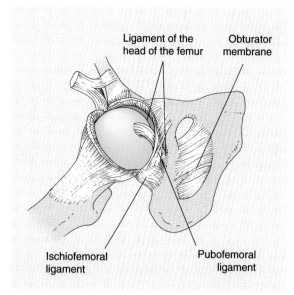

Figure 4.116 Right hip joint after the opening of the joint capsule.

follows the contact on the level of the gemellus superior in "listening," so that the entire leg rotates minimally, either outward or inward. This movement is followed until it stops, then the therapist attempts to slightly reinforce the counter-movement that occurs. At the same time, the contact with the fascia of the superior gemellus muscle is intensified as if the therapist's fingertips were trying to reach through the patient's pelvis in the direction of the ceiling.

The technique described above requires the independent use of both of the therapist's hands, and attention to the contact of the sole of the foot from the patient. If there is sufficient coordination between the therapist and the patient, it is possible for us to produce an indirect connection to the ligaments that surround the hip joint from the outside. In order to do so, it is important that we actually follow the rotation of the leg within only the most minimal spatial changes without inducing too much muscle activity. In the most favorable case, this allows us to achieve a three-dimensional division of the reinforcing ligaments of the joint capsule.

Treatment of the connective tissue cushion in the acetabular fossa and the ligament of the head of the femur

Patient Supine, both legs extended.

Therapist Sitting at the foot of the treatment table.

Contact The sole of the patient's foot presses gently against the therapist's sternum, the weight of the leg is resting on both of the therapist's hands; the therapist is using one palm to support the thigh from the posterior direction and the other hand to support the lower leg from the posterior direction.

Action While the therapist's sternum gently touches the sole of the foot, the therapist supports the lower leg and thigh from the posterior direction and follows rotations that occur between the two sections of the legs, which may take on a slight knock-kneed or bow-legged shape. It is important to follow the dominant pattern and, at the same time, maintain contact with the sole of the foot. As soon as the dominant pattern is manifest, the therapist gently pushes along the central line of the leg toward the hip joint. This push should be performed at the same time with the sternum against the sole of the foot and the supporting hands on the thigh and lower leg. At the moment at which the

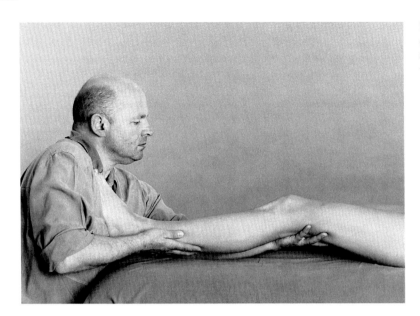

Figure 4.117   Treatment of the connective tissue cushion in the acetabular fossa and the ligament of the head of the femur.

resistance in the hip joint becomes obvious, the therapist guides the entire leg slightly in the medial direction, i.e. in the direction of the connective tissue cushion in the acetabular fossa and ligament of the head of the femur. The therapist thus presses the fovea of the head of the femur against the connective tissue cushion and against the ligament on the medial portion of the acetabulum. As soon as the therapist detects a counterforce, the therapist follows the tiny wave of pressure that manifests in the entire leg and thus allows a tiny expansion of the joint space and thus a redistribution of joint fluid.

This technique may be summarized in a simplified fashion as follows: the therapist guides the head of the femur in small steps farther into the joint socket until a slight counterpressure is felt. The therapist intensifies this counterpressure gradually with the feeling of the fingertips so that the head of the femur figuratively wanders out of the joint socket. Even though this is a minimal spatial change, its effect is lasting in terms of the distribution of joint fluid.

This is an effect of the connective tissue and ligament structure in the interior of the joint capsule. Because the goal of this treatment is a better distribution of joint fluid, it is essential that the shear force exerted by the therapist has

such a subtle effect that it reaches the interior of the joint capsule. Any rough, mechanical traction on the leg must be avoided because it would only lead to the movement of exterior layers and usually does not address the interior movement pattern in the capsule. If the technique described above is successful, the patient has a sensation as though the entire leg were wandering out of the hip in the distal direction and becoming longer.

Supplementary treatment techniques

The techniques described in the chapter on the lower extremity for the treatment of the fascia of the lower leg (treatment of the superficial layer of the crural fascia and treatment of the deep crural fascia) and of the band structures in the region of the ankle (treatment of the ankle) are suitable to supplement the treatment techniques described here. If restrictions in the movement of the pelvic organs can be felt on the side of the affected joint, treatment with the techniques described in detail by Jean-Pierre Barral and Paul Mercier is advisable (Barral and Mercier 2002).

The organs of the urogenital tract are particularly significant in this context, particularly the kidneys and bladder.

There is also one other starting point for treatment that deals with the nerves bordering the hip region. Barral and Croibier have developed techniques for the treatment of the peripheral nerves that go beyond the original visceral concept. These techniques appear to act directly on the connective tissue sheath layers of the nerves and therefore influence the forces acting between the nerve and its boundary surfaces. In the region of the hip joint, the technique mentioned above can be applied to the femoral and obturator nerves.

> A very efficient technique for the treatment of the obturator membrane may be found in Prat (1993: 7–33).

Chapter 5

Special joint techniques

5.1 VERTEBRAL JOINTS

Before treatment of vertebral and costal joints, the restriction of motion of the joint is first examined in the context of the small muscular and ligamentous units near the joint. Then we look for a possible connection between the restriction of movement and larger tissue layers or structures. In the case of the spine, we are concerned with the curvatures of the individual sections of the spine along with all of the structures in the region of the cervical, thoracic, and lumbar spine.

When performing this treatment in practice, the therapist must be able to use both hands and the individual fingers independently of one another so as to produce five or more contact points to the side of the spine with one hand. This plurality of contact points is necessary because only in this manner can we achieve an effect on tissue layers near the joint while keeping a large portion of the back in a position that facilitates treatment.

Treatment of motion restrictions of vertebral joints in the thoracic spine

Patient Supine, both legs extended.

Therapist Sitting at the head.

Contact The back of the patient's head rests on both of the therapist's forearms; the fingertips of both of the therapist's hands are touching the tissue to both sides of the affected joint.

Action   The weight of the therapist's forearms is transferred onto the treatment table in such a way that the flexion musculature of the forearms is as relaxed as possible and the back of the patient's head is resting on it as if on two soft pillows. The therapist now positions the fingertips of both hands on both sides of the blocked joint slightly below the transverse processes of both vertebrae. If the therapist's forearms are offset from one another on the treatment table, one hand will be able to reach somewhat farther downward than the other. It is crucial that the patient be relaxed, with the critical zone resting on the therapist's fingertips. The therapist supports the region of the thoracic spine in such a way that the habitual curvature of this section of the spine and back that is typical for every patient shows up. At the same time, the therapist uses "listening" to follow every movement, no matter how small, that is sensed in the movement-restricted joint. The therapist intensifies this movement tendency in the direction in which it can be felt most strongly and, in so doing, moves the joint more into its restriction. In the brief moment of this "wedging," the tactile sense of the therapist's fingertips concentrates on the pull of the soft tissue. The therapist gradually intensifies the contact in a very precise manner with these tissue units, which may be quite small, until a countermotion can be felt that guides the joint out of its blockage. In the case of a genuine fixation of the joint on both sides, this process may take approximately two to three minutes.

Treatment of costal vertebral joints in the mid-region of the thoracic spine

Patient   Sitting on a stool.

Therapist   Standing at the patient's side with one foot on the seat of the stool in order to support the elbow of the hand applying the treatment on the thigh.

Contact   Precisely below the affected rib and slightly lateral of the costotransverse articulation.

Action   The patient relaxes both hands and places them on the pectoral girdle without interlocking them. The therapist holds both of the patient's elbows so as to be able to guide the patient's upper body in passive rotation and lateral flexion. The therapist now examines how the tissue and the blocked joint in the area of fixation behave when the ribcage is rotated slightly to the left and right. For this treatment, it is important to prevent rotation to the side where the blockage is reflected. Instead, the therapist rotates the patient's upper body in the other direction while using the thumb to maintain the pressure in the tissue below the rib. It is important that the patient's upper body not be overextended in this process. It is crucial that the

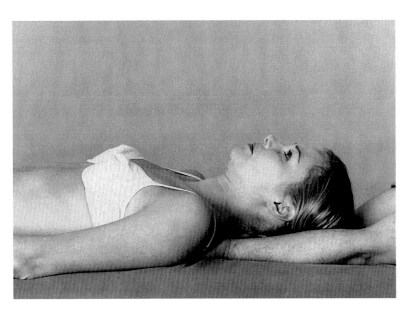

Figure 5.1   Treatment of motion restrictions of vertebral joints in the thoracic spine.

contact with the thumb remain very sensitive in order to sense precisely how the blockage changes with the lateral rotation. It is sometimes necessary to combine the lateral rotation with minimal lateral flexion of the thoracic spine.

A similar treatment technique with the patient lying down is recommended for the lower three ribs.

In the case of very increased tone in the musculature of the pectoral girdle, this technique cannot be successfully applied to the two upper costal vertebral joints. In such a case, the mobilization of the posterior scalene fascia or a direct joint manipulation is advisable.

Before applying this technique, it is advisable to first examine and, if necessary, treat the connection of the ribs to the sternum in the anterior region (see section 4.1, Treatment of the sternoclavicular connection). Under some circumstances, treatment should also extend to global tension patterns of the myofascial layers that are located in the retrosternal region (see section 4.1, Treatment of the sternum and the transversus thoracis). The transversus thoracis and, for the lower ribs, the uppermost segment of the transversus abdominis, which is directly adjacent to the transversus thoracis, are particularly significant here. Because the rib–vertebra connection is a double joint—the costotransverse articulation and the costovertebral articulation—and because tendons, ligaments, muscles, and membranes are attached to this joint in a wide variety of directions, this technique requires precise knowledge of the joint mechanism.

Treatment of the lower three costal vertebral joints

Patient   Supine, both legs extended.

Therapist   Standing at the level of the hips.

Contact   With both hands from the posterior direction in the region of the lower three ribs.

Action   The therapist surrounds the ribcage with both hands from the posterior direction, adapts the

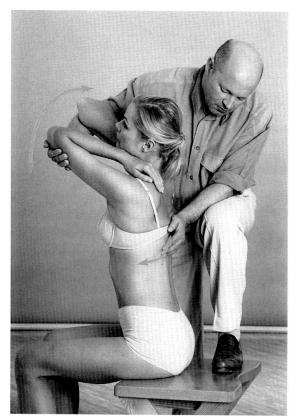

Figure 5.2   Treatment of costal vertebral joints in the middle region of the thoracic spine.

hands to the costal arch, and rotates the lower section of the chest cavity as a whole, first in one direction and then in the other. Below the fixated joint, the therapist's thumb reaches into the tissue from the lateral direction. While allowing this thumb contact to act as a wedge, the therapist rotates both halves of the thorax opposite one another in a tiny rotation, as if the body consisted of two self-contained cylinders in this area. It is important to perform the rotation of the two "cylinders" in such a way that the joint fixation of the ribs is reinforced until a countermovement manifests in the fixation, which the therapist uses to correct it.

Treatment of motion restrictions in the upper lumbar spine

Patient   Prone.

Therapist   Sitting next to the treatment table at the level of the abdomen.

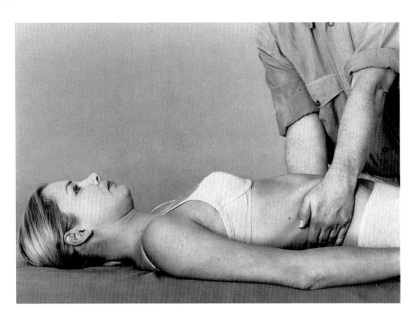

Figure 5.3 Treatment technique for the lower three costovertebral joints.

Contact   With one hand on both sides next to the sternum, in the region in which the fifth, sixth, and seventh ribs are connected to the sternum; at the same time, with the other hand and extended forearm supporting the thighs from the anterior direction.

Action   The therapist first places both hands in the initial position described above and then selects the contact in the region of the lower sternum as the fixed point and uses the fingertips and heel of the hand to press in the direction of the xiphoid process. This pressure should act inward, that is to say, influence the tension of both cupulas of the diaphragm and their ligamentous connection to the stomach and liver. The arm and hand that the therapist is using to support the thighs now perform a slight rotational motion to the left and right, which is then repeated several times in minimal steps. This causes a spatial displacement of the insertion of the psoas on the lesser trochanter. By this repeated subtle movement, which covers only a few millimeters, an induction of the flexion and extension of the psoas muscle occurs. Finally, the therapist rotates the patient's pelvis, which is moved as one unit, and legs against the fixed thoracolumbar transition.

If the therapist now applies the diagnostic principle of general "listening," the therapist will be able to sense the behavior of the joint fixation in the upper lumbar area in relation to the passively induced movement.

If performed precisely, this technique has the advantage that it includes prevertebral and posterior layers in the treatment at the same time. If the fixation of the upper lumbar vertebrae is more strongly pronounced on the left side, a variation of this technique is advisable: with one hand, the therapist grasps not the arch of the ribs and sternum, but rather the left section of the duodenum in the direction of Treitz's ligaments and uses a stretching impulse to guide it to its connection point on the upper lumbar spine and back again.

Decompression technique for the transition between the lower lumbar spine and sacrum

In the literature, there are numerous descriptions of techniques for treatment of the transition between the lumbar spine and sacrum. The technique described here is similar to techniques that are already known.[1]

Patient   Supine, both legs extended.

Therapist   Standing at the level of the thigh.

---

[1] For example, cf. the detailed descriptions in Upledger and Vredevoogd (1983: 141–2).

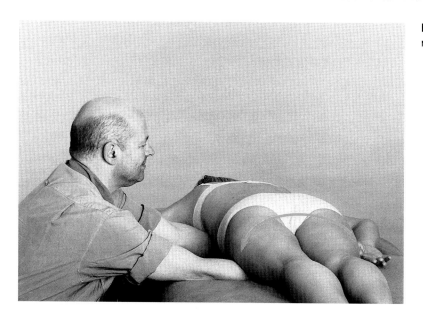

Figure 5.4 Treatment of motion restrictions in the upper lumbar spine.

Contact With the palm of one hand supporting the sacrum, with the fingertips just reaching the base of the sacrum, while the other hand creates a contact with the tissue layers near the joint on both sides of the lumbar spine at the level of the fourth and fifth lumbar vertebrae.

Action The therapist supports the sacrum with one hand, trying to adapt the shape of the palm to the individual shape of the posterior surface of the sacrum as best as possible. With the other hand, the therapist creates contact on both sides of the fourth and fifth lumbar vertebrae with the tissue layers of the lower back. This action is a specification of the technique that we have already learned in the treatment of curvature of the lumbar spine in its transition to the sacrum (see section 4.1, Treatment of lumbar lordosis at the transition to the pelvic cavity). First, the last lumbar vertebra and sacrum are compressed and, in so doing, we precisely trace any small rotation and lateral flexions movements that may occur between the bony units on our hands. Only when the tissue layers involved no longer provide resistance to us is the sacrum moved in the inferior direction out of its compression against the last lumbar vertebra.

Superficially regarded, this process first appears to be a simple relaxation technique. In reality, however, the relaxation of the musculature and the

major muscle layers is only the precondition for the actual treatment of the small muscular units and ligament and tendon units of this section of the body. In this context, it is of interest to observe that the iliolumbar ligament is first constructed as a muscular structure and does not turn into a purely ligamentous structure until an advanced age, approximately around the thirtieth year of life. If there is a compression between the fifth lumbar vertebra and the first sacral vertebra due to a general, very strongly pronounced muscle tone, the therapist can, without reservation, use the fingertips to apply a massive pull on the part of the lumbar fascia that runs between the sacrum and subdermis instead of the subtle traction on the sacrum in the inferior direction. In this regard, the technique is similar to Ida Rolf's "pelvic lift." [2]

Treatment of motion restrictions of the lower cervical spine

Patient Supine, both legs bent.

Therapist Sitting to the side at the head of the treatment table.

[2] The term "pelvic lift" also occurs in Sutherland (1990: 281–2).

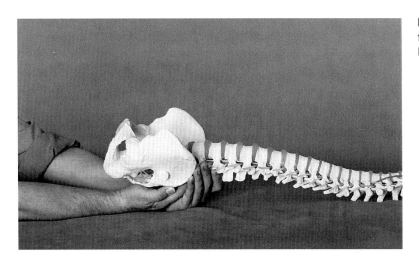

Figure 5.5 Decompression technique for the transition between the lower lumbar spine and sacrum.

Contact The therapist supports the back of one forearm and the back of the hand on the treatment table and places the four fingertips and tip of the thumb vertically around the spinous process of the first thoracic vertebra, supporting the occiput with the other hand.

Action With the position of the fingers and thumb around the upper thoracic vertebra described above, the therapist forms five support points more or less in the shape of a circle in the region of the lower section of the nuchal ligament, which begins at that point to connect to the fascia of the trapezius muscle. With the other hand, the therapist raises the patient's head somewhat and pushes it gently in the inferior direction, as if to push the entire cervical spine slightly into the ribcage. The contact around the first thoracic vertebra is maintained throughout this process, as if the therapist were trying to send all imaginable energy from the fingertips, through the patient's tissue, and in the direction of the ceiling. The therapist now begins to minimally move the head and neck alternately to the left and right in rotation and lateral flexion. Here, the therapist is gradually reducing the push in the inferior direction. In other words, the therapist is no longer pushing the cervical spine and neck into the upper chest cavity, but rather is accompanying the neck in the opposite, cranial direction. In so doing, the therapist allows every lateral movement of the neck, regardless of how minimal, while the supporting contact at the base of the skull remains very light and the

contact around the uppermost thoracic vertebra remains very firm.

If the restriction of movement in the vertebral segments described above is the result of a spasm-like, lasting flexion of the scalene group, the contact should be made between the upper ribs to which the scalene musculature is attached instead of around the first thoracic vertebra.

Treatment of the atlanto–occipital connection

There is such a variety of tissue layers in the short section between the axis, the atlas, and the base of the skull that it is not easy to decide where the force is originating that is ultimately causing a restriction of movement at the atlanto-occipital joints and, under some circumstances, fixating it on a lasting basis. At the transitional zone between the cervical spine and the head, quite literally all of the layers may be involved, beginning with the surface of the galea aponeurotica, which contains motor and sensory nerves, through the suboccipital musculature, into the interior of the vertebral canal and cranium through the dura. In addition, tension patterns from sections of the body located in the inferior direction can easily transfer onto the atlanto-occipital connection.

Restraint is advisable in the case of unilateral joint fixations because they rarely have a local origin; rather, they arise from the various compressional and tensional conditions in both halves of the body

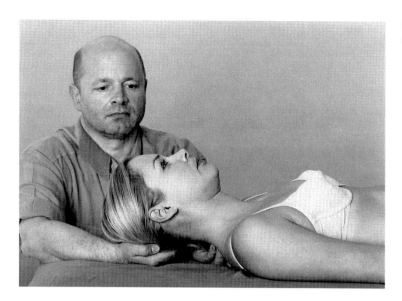

Figure 5.6   Treatment of motion restrictions of the lower cervical spine.

below the neck. However, it is also true for bilateral, genuine joint fixations on the occipital condyle that the dominant tensile forces can originate at a greater distance from the joint, for example, at the joint between the coccyx and sacrum. If the coccyx is chronically displaced in the anterior direction and is limited in its mobility relative to the sacrum, then the dura comes under a large amount of tensional forces over its entire course into the foramen magnum. It is possible that the tensional conditions are also changing in the large anterior longitudinal ligament, which is directly connected to the atlanto-occipital membrane. In any event, it can be seen over and over in practice that a mobilization of the coccyx leads to a direct and very long-lasting relief of the transition between the atlas and the base of the skull. Then we must make only a minimal subsequent correction at the atlanto-occipital transition.

If we apply our treatment directly to the region of the joints at the head of the atlas, the relatively small muscles that run in the posterior direction are important.

Here, it should be taken into account that the obliquus capitis inferior, the rectus capitis major, and the rectus capitis posterior minor all run diagonally to the middle line of the neck at different angles of incline. The angle of incline is most pronounced in the rectus capitis posterior minor, which runs almost vertically between the posterior atlantic tubercule and the internal third of the

nuchal line. This small muscle, which appears to have a fascial connection to the dura, is of central significance to treatment practice because it can cause a massive compression of the atlanto-cranial joints due to its almost vertical course.

However, in the case of chronic joint fixation, it is certainly not only the tone pattern of one individual muscle or muscle group that plays a deciding role. Rather, it is the cooperation of the various tissues that changes the mobility of a joint on a lasting basis. Therefore, the following technique combines direct tissue contact with a type of positioning known from Jones 1981.

Patient   Supine, both legs bent.

Therapist   Sitting at the head.

Contact   With the fingertips of both hands on the atlanto-occipital transition, if possible.

Action   It is fundamental for this technique that the therapist first exaggerate the joint position that is typical of the fixation. The therapist supports the patient's occiput very gently, then reaches directly below the base of the skull toward the atlanto-occipital membrane after having moved the joint laterally and rotated it corresponding to its fixation. Now, the therapist's sternum pushes directly against the top of the skull in such a way that the joint position is reinforced. In so doing, the therapist pushes the foremost part of the fingertips of the index and

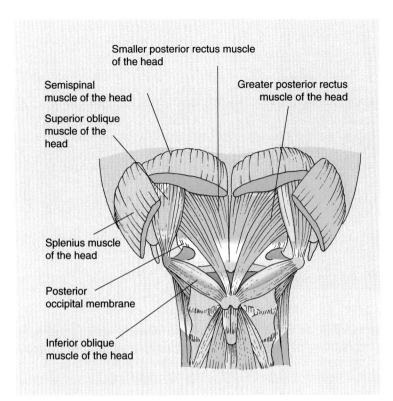

Smaller posterior rectus muscle of the head

Semispinal muscle of the head

Superior oblique muscle of the head

Greater posterior rectus muscle of the head

Splenius muscle of the head

Posterior occipital membrane

Inferior oblique muscle of the head

Figure 5.7   Deep muscles in the region of the posterior section of the neck.

middle fingers toward the more strongly fixated side in the direction of the joint connection and maintains a "melting contact" with the tissue there. The therapist pays the greatest attention to every small change in tone at this point. As soon as the therapist's fingertips are able to sense an increase in radiated heat or a reduction in tone of the small muscular units, then the therapist slowly rotates the head and neck back into their normal position.

Compared with direct joint manipulation, the technique described above has the advantage that it has a very gentle and protective effect on the tissue layers. Moreover, it is advantageous that the combination of positioning the joint and applying a direct effect on the tissue layers allows us to reach the myofascial units, membranes, tendons, and ligaments at the same time. If we omit the push against the roof of the skull and vary the hand position accordingly, this technique can also be applied effectively in the region of the middle cervical vertebral joints.

Treatment of the membrane connections between the axis, atlas, and occipital bone

Patient   Supine, both legs extended.

Therapist   Sitting to the side at the level of the neck.

Contact   Supporting the tissue covering the posterior arch and transverse process of the atlas from the posterior direction with the thumb and index finger; the other hand supports the occiput and its fingertips maintain contact just below the base of the skull.

Action   The primary weight of the head is transferred onto the supporting hand on the base of the skull; only part of the weight of the neck is resting on the contact point at the posterior arch of the atlas. The therapist gradually lifts the atlas slightly in the anterior direction, specifically in such a way that the vertebra moves minimally along the articular fascia. While doing so, we are guided by imagining that we are moving the anterior arch of the axis onto the anterior part of the pons of the occiput so that a relaxation occurs in the anterior portion of the

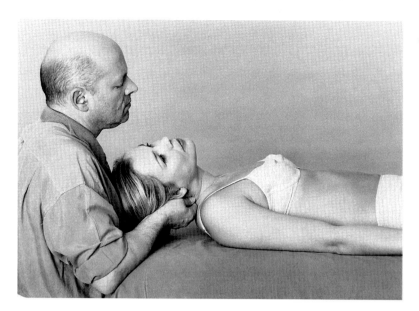

Figure 5.8 Treatment of the atlanto-occipital connection.

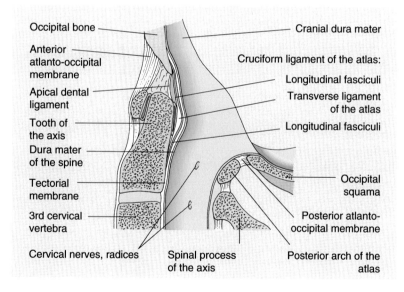

Occipital bone

Anterior
atlanto-occipital
membrane

Apical dental
ligament

Tooth of
the axis

Dura mater
of the spine

Tectorial
membrane

3rd cervical
vertebra

Cervical nerves, radices

Spinal process
of the axis

Cranial dura mater

Cruciform ligament of the atlas:

Longitudinal fasciculi

Transverse ligament
of the atlas

Longitudinal fasciculi

Occipital
squama

Posterior atlanto-
occipital membrane

Posterior arch of the
atlas

Figure 5.9 Medial section of the joints of the head.

atlanto-occipital membrane. Once the therapist is able to sense the relaxation, the therapist first follows only the atlas with "listening"—the occiput remains a fixed point—then the therapist follows the occiput in any small movements that may occur. As soon as these movements abate, the therapist changes the contact to the second cervical vertebra while continuing to support the patient's occiput. The therapist now attempts to affect the tectorial membrane and the short piece of the spinal dura mater that runs between the occiput and the axis.

For this purpose, it is necessary to twist the occiput and axis minimally opposite one another while "listening," finally to guide them together and wait for the shear effect that occurs in the small intermediate area between the occiput, atlas, and axis.

Treatment of the iliosacral joints using the ligament and membrane connections of the pelvic cavity

Patient Prone.

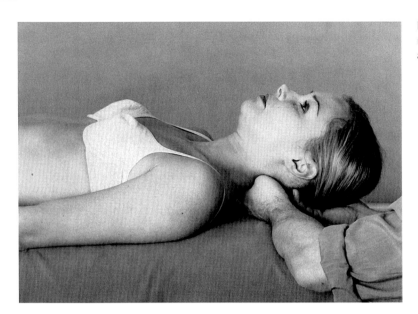

Figure 5.10 Treatment of the membrane connections between the axis, atlas, and occipital bone.

Therapist   Standing at the level of the hips.

Contact   With one hand on the sacrum and the other hand transverse to it from the anterior direction slightly below the navel.

Action   The therapist tests the mobility between the organs and the sacrum by exerting vertical pressure in the anterior direction precisely on the second segment of the sacrum. The therapist observes whether this pressure arrives at the anterior hand placed on the abdomen. If this is not the case, it is a sign that strong tensions exist between the sacrum and the organs located anterior to it. In this case, the therapist uses the anterior hand to lift the entire abdominal cavity in the posterior direction toward the sacrum. During this movement, the contact with the posterior hand on the sacrum is maintained. The therapist subsequently allows the abdominal cavity to sink back a few millimeters in the anterior direction and follows the movement with "listening." If the therapist's hand rotates in one direction, the therapist follows this movement to its end in order to exert posterior pressure in the direction of the sacrum. The contact with the other hand on the sacrum is maintained unabated during this process; its quality should be slightly elastic. In this manner, the ligamentous connection between the cervix and sacrum becomes more mobile. This in turn improves the mobility of the neck of the uterus. The forces that may be fixating the sacrum from the anterior direction find an improved equilibrium.

Mobilization of the inferior section of the iliosacral joint

Patient   Supine, both legs extended.

Therapist   Standing at the level of the thighs.

Contact   One hand supports the region of the upper lumbar spine from the posterior direction and the other hand supports the sacrum, with the palm touching the lower part of the sacrum in order to guarantee that the fingertips can be moved laterally.

Action   The supporting hand in the region of the lumbar spine reinforces the lordotic curvature. This causes a general reduction in tension in the major extensors of the back. We ensure that the patient is not "holding" the position, but rather that the weight of the patient's entire body is being transferred into our hands. By reinforcing the lordotic curvature, the pelvis is tilted slightly in the anterior direction. We follow this movement with the hand supporting the sacrum. We now observe how the sacrum behaves with regard to the reduction in tone of the musculature in the region of the lower lumbar spine. The pulling effect of the ligaments will become far more tangible. Under certain circumstances, the sacrum may tilt in a diagonal direction, rotate slightly, or move in a clockwise or counterclockwise direction. We first register the direction in which the sacrum is being pulled or pushed and use our hand to feel both lateral edges

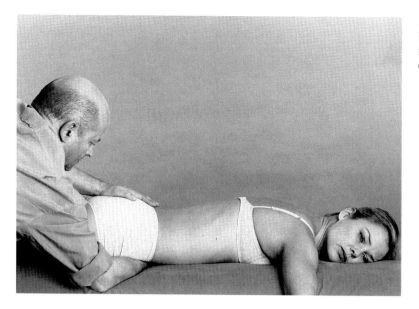

Figure 5.11 Treatment of the iliosacral joints using the ligament and membrane connections of the pelvic cavity.

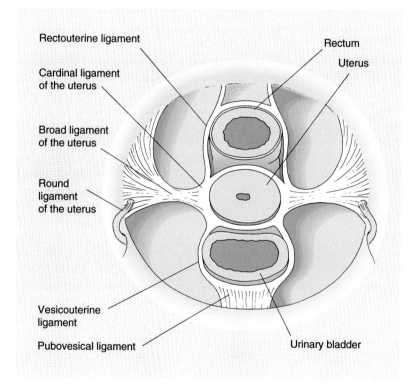

Rectouterine ligament

Cardinal ligament of the uterus

Broad ligament of the uterus

Round ligament of the uterus

Vesicouterine ligament

Pubovesical ligament

Rectum

Uterus

Urinary bladder

Figure 5.12 Ligamentous connection between the bladder, neck of the uterus, and rectum.

of the sacrum very precisely. We concentrate entirely on detecting whether we can feel one individual segment of the bone as conspicuously rigid. This is frequently the point at which a ligament with a high concentration of fibers exercises pull.

However, sometimes it is also the region of the origin of the anterior piriform muscle. Under certain circumstances, we can feel a type of rigidity on the posterior section of the lower joint connection itself, which I presume comes from the lasting tension of

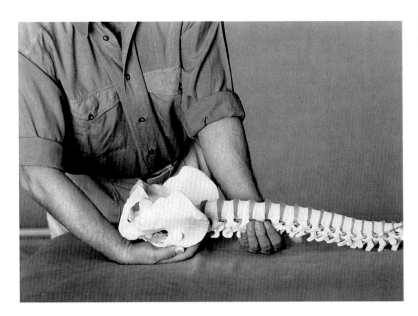

Figure 5.13   Mobilization of the inferior section of the iliosacral joint.

the sacroiliac ligament, which is interwoven with the lumbar fascia. Some skill is required to keep the lumbar region in a lordosis to support the lower part of the sacrum with the palm and use one or two fingertips to produce contact on the connection of the ligament or the tendinous insertion of a muscle on the periosteum as if we wanted to make this connection "melt." If this technique is performed precisely, the sacrum "swims" into a normal relationship to the two ilia.

In order to check the result of treatment, it is advisable to have the patient stand up and walk a few steps. Then the patient should lie supine again, the therapist lifts the patient's spine into an increased lordosis, allows the sacrum to tilt slightly in the anterior direction, and determines whether the unfavorable pull effect of myofascial units and ligaments has been reduced. Ideally, the sacrum will now exhibit an intensified tilt without escaping more to the side or making rotational motions.

5.2   TREATMENT OF INTERVERTEBRAL DISK PROTRUSIONS

In spite of great progress in imaging processes, it is not always easy to decide whether the protrusion shown on an MRI image is actually responsible for the discomfort the patient is suffering. From orthopedic practice, we know numerous examples of a drastic protrusion being visible on the MRI image but no dysfunction being associated with it and the patient being free of discomfort.

With this fact in mind, it is worthwhile to attempt to treat disk problems manually, even if it is not entirely certain that the dysfunction is actually originating from the intervertebral disk. Manual treatment should be applied only if we can rule out the danger of neurological damage—and even then under neurological supervision.

The techniques below are particularly suited for application in the region of the lumbar and cervical spine. It is fundamentally necessary for the patient to be positioned such that compensatory muscle spasms are reduced to the greatest extent possible and the acute symptoms are alleviated for the moment. The therapist should avoid any abrupt manual intervention and only conduct shear, rotational, and tilt movements slowly and in small degrees in order to avoid additional irritation of the affected nerve.

Treatment of intervertebral disk protrusions in the region of the lower lumbar spine

This technique is suitable for the treatment of lateral protrusions. In most cases, it has been shown in practice that the patient should be positioned on the unaffected side. This allows the intervertebral disk to sink back somewhat into the intervertebral

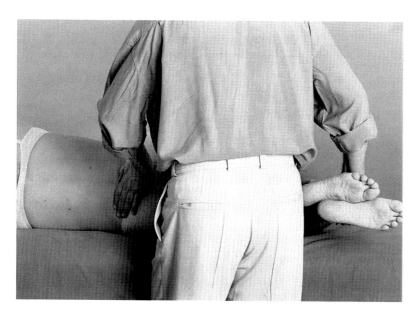

Figure 5.14 Treatment of intervertebral disk protrusions in the region of the lower lumbar spine.

space under the weight of its gelatinous filling as soon as the pressure from the two adjacent vertebrae has been reduced.

Patient Lying on one side, legs bent.

Therapist Standing at the level of the hips facing the patient's back.

Contact With one flat palm in the region of the lower lumbar spine at the transition to the sacrum; the other hand surrounds both ankles from the anterior side.

Action The therapist uses the palm to precisely sense the motion behavior of the vertebrae in the critical zone. With the other hand, the therapist surrounds both of the patient's ankles and gently pulls the patient's bent legs in the posterior direction in order to change the kinked transition between the lower lumbar spine and the sacrum into a "soft" curvature.

In the second treatment step, the therapist's thigh is positioned for support below the patient's lower leg in such a way that the tilt of the right side of the pelvis around the hip axis in the anterior direction is somewhat more pronounced and the right side of the pelvis rotates slightly in the direction of the center line of the body. With the other hand, the therapist maintains flat contact in the lateral region of the lower ribs and pushes the

intraperitoneal organs diagonally in the anterocranial direction toward the diaphragm. This causes a slight release of pressure between the intra- and retroperitoneal space, while the positioning of the patient reinforces the stricture in the critical intervertebral space. The therapist now attempts to use "listening" to precisely detect the behavior of the vertebrae located above and below the herniation. I assume that, in so doing, we are able to influence the fiber pulls of the intervertebral disk ring in the moment of an indirect release of pressure.

In addition to "listening," we also need the permanent feedback from the patient regarding the pressure or release of pressure on the critically affected nerve in order to regulate this technique. The angle of pelvic tilt and extent of induced pelvic rotation are crucial.

If the application of this technique causes the pain situation to spontaneously improve, it is helpful to allow the patient to rest for a while longer in the treatment position.

This technique is also suitable for treating multiple protrusions in the region of the lower lumbar spine.

Treatment of lumbar intervertebral disk protrusions in the retromedial region according to Barral

Patient Prone.

Therapist Standing, one knee bent on the treatment table.

Contact The thigh of the therapist's bent leg supports the patient's legs slightly in the cranial direction above the knees and, at the same time, the therapist reaches around both legs in this region.

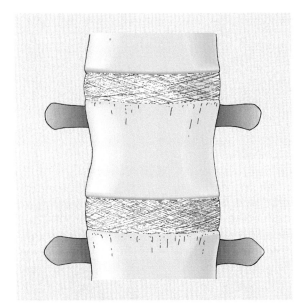

Figure 5.15 Fiber orientation of the fibrous ring of an intervertebral disk in the region of the lumbar spine.

Action The therapist positions the patient prone carefully enough to avoid additional nerve irritation. The therapist then places one hand in the region of the affected segment of the back. The contact should be loose enough to allow the most subtle "listening." The goal of the position is to create a "soft" lordosis instead of the kink characterized by compression between the fifth lumbar vertebra and first sacral segment or between the fourth and fifth lumbar vertebrae.

> Care should be taken if a spondylolisthesis is present with a long-term positional displacement in the anterior direction. In this case, it is advisable to support the abdominal cavity from the anterior direction and slide the peritoneum, including the retroperitoneal layers, slightly toward the critical segments in the posterior direction.

The therapist now uses a slight rotational movement of the thigh supporting the patient's legs to lift the patient's legs minimally and rotate the legs slightly to the left and to the right so that this movement is transmitted to the pelvis. The therapist accompanies this process with "listening" using the contact hand in the region of the critical lumbar

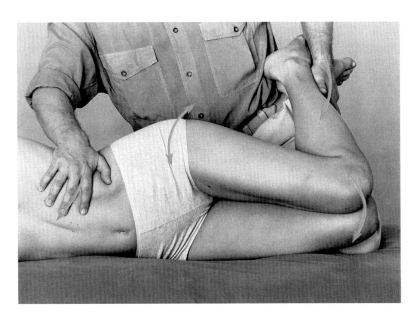

Figure 5.16 Treatment of intervertebral disk protrusions in the region of the lower lumbar spine, second treatment step.

segment. Rotation by rotation, the therapist relieves the intervertebral disk under pressure or, more precisely, the various components of the organism at the level of the intervertebral disk. Following with "listening," the therapist provides a minimal push in the anterior direction and, in so doing, allows the contents of the intervertebral disk to sink farther in the anterior direction under the influence of gravity and the protrusion of the membrane being compressed in the retromedial direction to subside. The therapist subsequently allows the patient to slide out of the treatment position slowly and carefully.

Treatment of lateral intervertebral disk protrusions in the region of the neck

Patient Supine, both legs bent.

Therapist Sitting at the head.

Contact One hand supports the neck and the base of the skull from the posterior direction while the fingertips of the other hand produce a contact at the level of the costovertebral joints between the second and third ribs.

Action The therapist supports the neck and head lifted at the same angle as the general curvature that is present in the patient's cervical spine. If the tendency toward hyperextension is present, the therapist supports it without reinforcing it too much. If there is a tendency toward a pronounced lordosis, the therapist should support this form as well without exaggerating it. In both cases, it is crucial that the therapist avoid placing a mechanical pull on the cervical spine in the cranial direction. Any pulling effect on the exterior myofascial layers of the neck should be omitted as well because such an effect could lead to a counterreaction of small muscular units in the deep layers and thus cause an unfavorable compression of the affected segment. The therapist holds the other hand between the upper ribs on both sides of the spine in such a way that the fingertips are placed precisely between the second and third ribs and the costovertebral joints to the left and right of the spine come to rest on the therapist's fingertips. The therapist now performs various small rotational and lateral movements until a neck position has been achieved that is pleasant and relaxing for the patient. If radiating pain is present in the arm, it will be reduced at the moment at which correct positioning is achieved. While the therapist maintains this position, the contact with one hand on the tissue that covers the costovertebral joints from the posterior direction is intensified. The therapist's other hand now follows with "listening" and the therapist attempts to maintain the most precise possible contact with the tissue below and above the affected intervertebral disk. As soon as a change in tone manifests in this region, the therapist reduces the intensity of the

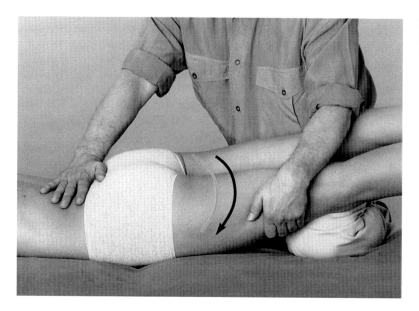

Figure 5.17 Treatment of lumbar intervertebral disk protrusions in the retromedial region according to Barral.

contact on the neck and, at the same time, directs tactile perception toward the minimal movement that manifests in both vertebrae above and below the affected intervertebral disk and accompanies both bones in this movement, which reduces the compression on the intervertebral disk.

Treatment variation for strongly pronounced lateral intervertebral disk protrusions in the neck region

The technique described above, with the patient lying supine, does not always yield the desired treatment result in cases of pronounced lateral protrusion. In such cases, it is advisable to apply this technique while the patient is lying on one side. It is important that the patient lies on the side that is not affected and that the patient's head is supported by a pillow.

Patient   Lying on the side contralateral to the herniation.

Therapist   Sitting at the head.

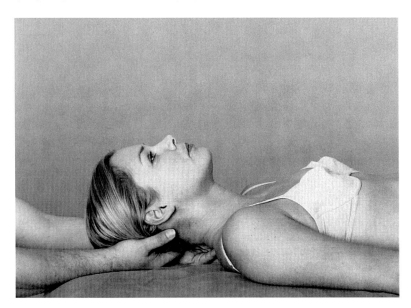

Figure 5.18   Treatment of lateral intervertebral disks protrusions in the region of the neck.

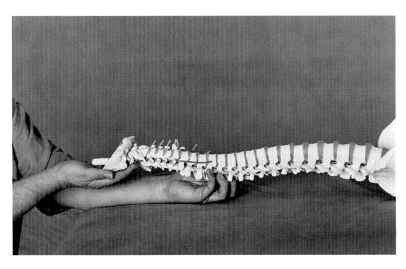

Figure 5.19   Hand position.

Contact   The therapist supports the patient's head from the side; the index and middle fingers of the other hand are located slightly cranially to the clavicle.

Action   The therapist now uses the two fingers to make a direct contact to the brachial plexus on the side of the protrusion. The therapist exerts a slight pull on the perineurial sheath as if to gently pluck the string of a guitar. While doing so, the therapist raises the patient's head slightly in lateral flexion and rotation. Then the lateral flexion and rotation of the neck is gradually scaled back to its starting position so that a pull occurs on the perineurial sheath of the brachial plexus. The interaction of the positioning of the neck and pull effect on the nerve itself decompresses the intervertebral foramen.

Treatment of retromedial intervertebral disk protrusions in the region of the cervical spine

Patient   Prone, with the head and neck extending past the head of the treatment table.

Therapist   Sitting at the head.

Contact   With one hand supporting the frontal bone and with the other hand inferior to both clavicles in the region of the subclavius muscle.

Action   It is important to ensure that the therapist completely supports the patient's head when the patient assumes the position. This prevents any unpleasant pull effect in the critical region of the neck. The therapist holds the complete weight of the head in one hand and should under no circumstances use the weight of the head to pull the neck in the cranial direction or, conversely, bend the head in the dorsal direction. Rather, the therapist takes the head in the hand in such a way that the curvature of the cervical spine and the myofascial layers in the interior of the neck are in such a position as to relieve the critical segment. Feedback from the patient regarding the radiating pain is essential to this treatment as well. The therapist attempts to select the position of the neck and head in such a way that the acute pain is reduced somewhat or, in the most favorable case, disappears entirely. The position in which this occurs is the position that must be maintained. The therapist can find this position by applying supportive force on both sides in the region of the subclavius muscle while the therapist's other hand moves the cervical spine above the head in the most minimal lateral flexion and rotation movements. This movement should be gradually repeated to the left and right while the head and neck are guided minimally in the anterior direction. In my experience, the impression arises after a certain amount of time

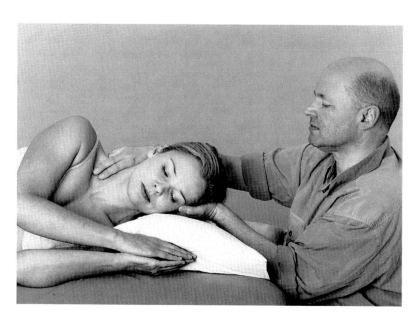

Figure 5.20 Treatment variation for strongly pronounced lateral intervertebral disk protrusions in the neck region.

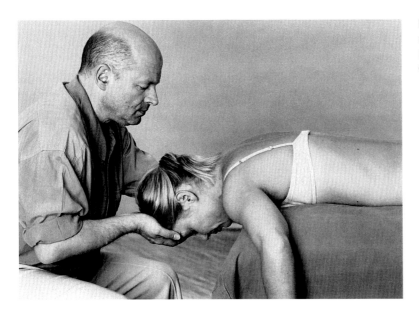

Figure 5.21 Treatment of retromedial intervertebral disk protrusions in the region of the cervical spine.

that the patient's head is resting more heavily in the therapist's hand. This is a sign of reduction in tone of the large extensors of the back and a relaxation of the scalene group. As soon as the therapist is able to feel a slight shear force in the direction of the top of the skull—in other words, as soon as the neck is trying to push slightly in the cranial direction out of the transitional point on the thorax—the therapist follows this movement. In so doing, it is important to ensure that we actually only follow this movement and avoid any major pull effect on the outer layers of the neck.

This technique has proven itself even in the case of massive displacements of the protrusion of the intervertebral disk in the posterior direction in the vertebral canal. As mentioned above, any mechanical extension of the neck must be avoided in applying this technique. The treatment result will manifest only if the therapist is able to keep the critical zone, i.e. the two vertebrae that are compressing the affected intervertebral disk, in a somewhat suspended state, causing the intervertebral disk, which has been relieved of the pressure, to be moved back slightly out of the vertebral canal in the anterior direction by

the force of gravity. In serious cases, the entire treatment process can extend over approximately 20 minutes. Within this time, it should be possible to relax the neck layer by layer without mechanical extension in order to ultimately move the intervertebral disk by a slight induction of movement in the dura and spinal cord. Under no circumstances may the therapist release the patient's head and, after the technique has been completed, the therapist should carefully guide the patient to lie on one side while supporting the patient's head, and finally guide the patient to a sitting position.

Treatment of intervertebral disk protrusions in the region of the thoracic spine

Intervertebral disk problems in the region of the thoracic spine are encountered far more rarely than in the region of the lumbar or cervical spine. Because the thoracic spine is relatively stable, the treatment situation is difficult. However, because the surgical options are usually complicated and associated with a high level of risk, a careful attempt at manual treatment is worthwhile in any event.

The technique I describe is based on Barral's observation that it is possible to exert a pull on the

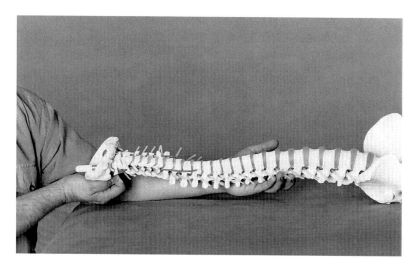

Figure 5.22 Treatment of intervertebral disk protrusions in the region of the thoracic spine.

dura as a whole beginning from the occiput. This pull should come into effect at the moment at which the cranium appears to become more filled with cerebrospinal fluid.

Patient Supine, both legs extended.

Therapist Sitting at the head.

Contact With one hand providing support on both sides at the level of the ninth thoracic vertebra and with the palm of the other hand on the occiput and its fingertips slightly below the base of the skull.

Action The therapist supports the back at the level of the ninth thoracic vertebra, i.e. at the point where the vertebral canal is particularly narrow. The therapist's fingertips are guided below the occiput as near as possible in the direction of the foramen magnum and the therapist attempts to transmit a pull effect onto the interior of the vertebral canal. In other words, the point is not to pull on the exterior on the neck or spine as a whole, but rather for the pull force to be transmitted by way of the attachment of the dura to the foramen magnum all the way into the interior of the vertebral canal, i.e. to the dura mater and the spinal cord. Using this pull effect, the therapist now creates a subtle contact with the segment inside which the protrusion is present. It is important to subtly modify the direction and extent of the pull in such a way that the compressive forces acting on the intervertebral disk change.

Applying this technique with two people increases its chances of success. The treatment assistant contacts the dura by way of its attachment on the second segment of the sacrum while the therapist contacts the foramen magnum in a manner similar to the one described above.

5.3 THE SACROCOCCYGEAL JOINT

A.T. Still, the founder of osteopathy, attached great significance to the coccyx and described the correction of movement restrictions at the sacrococcygeal joint. Ida Rolf, founder of the Rolfing Method, also assigned a prominent role to the coccyx in the course of the sixth of ten treatments in her basic treatment series. Recently, the coccyx has received renewed attention, primarily from Barral's practical research on visceral manipulation. This is certainly no coincidence because the effects of a motion-restricted sacrococcygeal joint can be seen in a particularly drastic fashion in the visceral region. Dysfunctions of the vesical sphincter, movement restrictions in or even sinking (ptosis) of the kidneys, movement restrictions at the ligamentous environment of the cervix and prostate—all of these phenomena can be better understood on the basis of the stabilizing role of the coccyx.

The significance of the coccyx as the stabilizing element of the lower pelvic cavity

In light of modern imaging techniques, the sacrococcygeal joint appears at first glance to be an

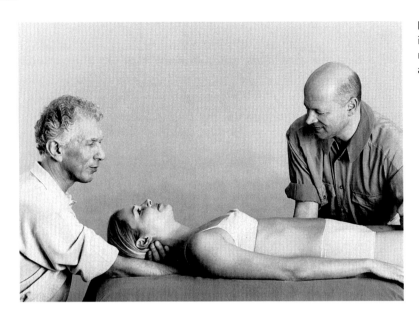

Figure 5.23 Treatment of intervertebral disk protrusions in the region of the thoracic spine by the author and Harvey Burns.

inessential appendage of the sacrum. Upon closer examination, however, although it is given little consideration in manual medicine, this joint proves itself to be one of the key points of the spine.

On the radiographic image taken from the sagittal direction, the coccyx is recognizable as a process of the sacrum that can display a quite varied individual angle of incline relative to the sacrum. If this angle of incline manifests itself in the form of a kink that is clearly visible in the radiographic image, this may be a sign of a restriction of movement between the sacrum and coccyx. This sign is not entirely absolute because the radiographic image provides only a momentary picture of the position of the bone. Manual tests are required to determine whether a reduction in normal mobility, which should be at least 15 degrees, is actually present.

For example, if the coccyx is fixated in the anterior direction, i.e. the range of motion between the coccyx and sacrum is considerably less than 15 degrees, then the distance between the origin and insertion of this muscle group is reduced as well and a reduction in muscle tone occurs. This process alters the pressure conditions in the pelvic cavity and thus influences the normal mobility of the organs.

The coccyx also plays a significant role with regard to the lower extremity because the large fascial sheaths of the semitendinosus and semimembranosus muscles have a direct connection to the ligaments and tendons that transition into the coccyx at the lowest edge of the sacrum.

Anatomy of the coccyx and adjacent structures

The coccyx has numerous variations in its bony structure. The number of bone segments can vary greatly (up to six units): in some cases, it is very long, but it can also be short and broad. These differences originate during embryonic development. As a rule, until the beginning of the second month, an embryo has a regular caudal process which the neural tube fills with the chorda, intestine, and mesoderm. During the second month of embryonic development, a reabsorption of this process gradually occurs.

The coccyx is connected in the cranial direction to the fifth segment of the sacrum by the sacrococcygeal synchondrosis. Both joint processes of the coccyx that point upward are connected by way of the articular sacrococcygeal ligament at this lowest segment of the sacrum here as well.

On the inferior side and in the deep layer of the pelvic floor, the coccyx is the insertion for the three

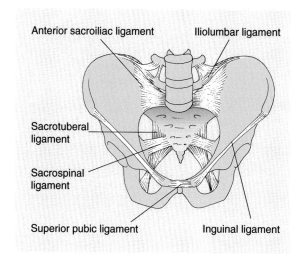

Figure 5.24   Pelvic bones and ligamentous apparatus of the male from the anterior direction.

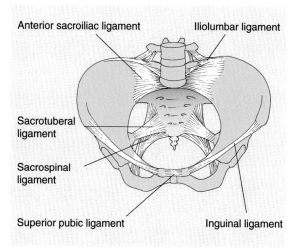

Figure 5.25   Pelvic bones and ligamentous apparatus of the female from the anterior direction.

muscular fascicles of the levator ani muscle: the iliococcygeal, pubococcygeal, and puborectal muscles. The exterior of this deep layer is surrounded by the gluteus maximus muscle, from which individual fascial fibers reach to the periosteum of the coccyx. The periosteum of the coccyx continues in a ligamentous fashion as the anococcygeal ligament and forms a bridge in the anterior direction to the external sphincter muscle of the anus.

The myofascial tension pattern of the musculature inserted at the coccyx plays an important role for the mobility of the coccyx. The massive fixation of the sacrococcygeal joint occurs in combination with the pull forces of the ligamentous and tendinous connections between the sacrum and coccyx, the coccyx and ischial tuberosity, and the coccyx and the spine of the ischium.

For the normal joint connection, it is characteristic for the sacrum to transition into the adjacent coccyx without a kink and for the coccyx to be harmoniously curved in and of itself without segmental kinks. Experience shows us that this normal joint connection may be found in only one-third of patients. The majority of patients have at one time or another fallen on the coccyx with grave consequences. For this reason, an examination should always be performed using one of the tests below, even in patients who do not complain of any symptoms in this region.

Examination

Examination of the pull effect of the coccyx fixated in the anterior direction on the lowest segment of the sacrum

Patient   Supine, both legs extended, arms resting next to the torso.

Therapist   Standing to the side at the level of the thighs.

Contact   With one palm on the sacrum from the posterior direction.

Action   As soon as the patient relaxes the superficial gluteal musculature, the sacrum will lower into the therapist's hand. It is important to relax the palm of the hand performing the test so that it can adapt precisely to the shape of the sacrum. In order to evaluate the sacrococcygeal joint, it is necessary to direct our tactile attention to the lowermost section of the sacrum. If the coccyx is displaced spatially in the anterior direction, the lowermost segment of the sacrum (fifth sacral vertebra) will feel rigid. It will be possible to move it only a very little way into the adjacent tissue layers. The sacrum feels as if the first through fourth sacral vertebrae have a "softer" bone structure than the fifth segment. This is a sign of past injury to the joint. The coccyx, which is held in the anterior direction by

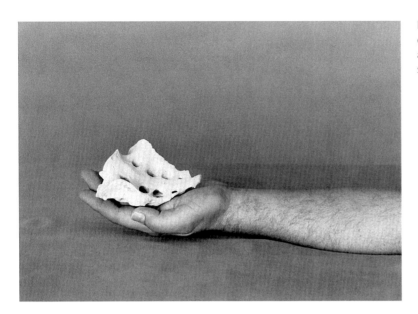

Figure 5.26   Examination of the pull effect of the coccyx fixated in the anterior direction on the lowest segment of the sacrum.

ligaments, has exerted a massive pull on the posterior fasciae of the deep posterior sacrococcygeal ligament over a long period of time and has caused more density of fibers there.

> This joint test gives us information as to whether the anterior displacement of the coccyx is manifesting in the posterior ligaments and tendons and extensions of the lumbar fascia. This test is not suitable for displacements of the coccyx that occurred only a few days ago.

Examination of anterior fixation of the coccyx and its displacement in the anterior direction

Patient   Sitting on the treatment table; the table should be adjusted to a sufficient height that the feet are dangling and are not in contact with the floor.

Therapist   Standing behind the patient, one knee supported on the treatment table.

Contact   With the index and middle fingers of one hand precisely touching the coccyx from below.

Action   The patient sits comfortably on the treatment table without the feet being in contact with

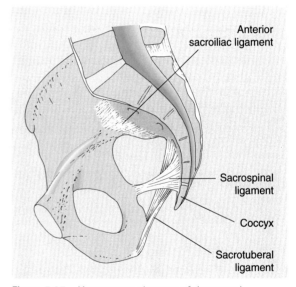

Figure 5.27   Ligamentous elements of the normal sacrococcygeal joint from the sagittal direction.

the floor; the patient's posture should be relaxed and not too straight. The therapist now touches the transition between the sacrum and coccyx and guides the index and middle fingers in the anterior direction until both fingers are precisely below the coccyx. In the case of an anterior displacement, the therapist now carefully applies upward pressure to the coccyx in order to determine whether the coccyx allows an elastic movement of 15–30 degrees

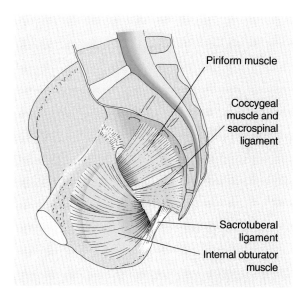

Figure 5.28   Muscles and ligaments of the normal sacrococcygeal joint from the sagittal direction.

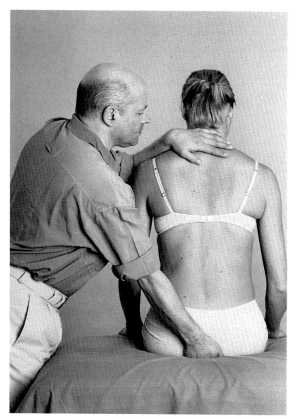

Figure 5.29   Examination of anterior fixation of the coccyx and its displacement in the anterior direction.

relative to the lower segment of the sacrum. If this movement is restricted, the patient will in most cases feel an intense pain on the joint.

As a rule, the anterior displacement and/or fixation of the coccyx is combined with a lateral displacement and/or fixation. For diagnosis, it is necessary to observe the sacrococcygeal joint during lateral flexion of the torso.

Examination of lateral fixation during lateral flexion of the torso

Patient   Sitting on the treatment table as described in the previous test.

Therapist   Standing behind the patient with one knee supported on the table.

Contact   With the index and middle fingers between the coccyx and ischial tuberosity on the right and left sides.

Action   The patient sits on the treatment table as in the preceding test. The therapist first touches both sides of the intermediate space between the coccyx and ischial tuberosity. In the case of a lateral fixation, the intermediate space will be constricted on one side. In a few cases, this sign can be misleading, namely when the constriction is caused not by the displaced coccyx, but rather by an unusual bone shape of the ischium. For this reason, it is necessary to verify the test result during lateral flexion of the torso.

In the case of normal joint function, the coccyx will move to the other side in the first phase of lateral movement so as to come over the central line to the flexion side of the torso. During the lateral bending, the patient's weight should be allowed to rest in both ischii.

If a lateral fixation is present on the right side, the intermediate space on the right side between the coccyx and ischial tuberosity will hardly change to the right. While the torso is in lateral flexion, the coccyx cannot move to the left in the first flexion phase. If a lateral fixation is present on the left side, the intermediate space on the right side between the coccyx and ischial tuberosity will hardly change to the left and the coccyx will not change to the right in the first lateral flexion phase.

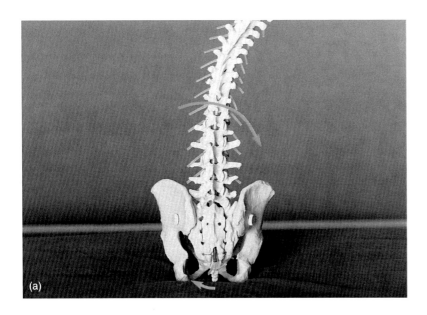

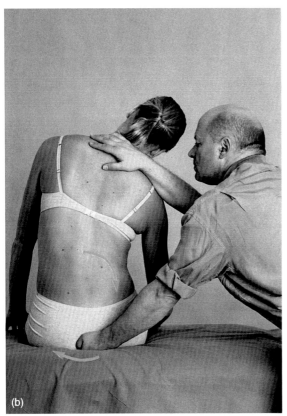

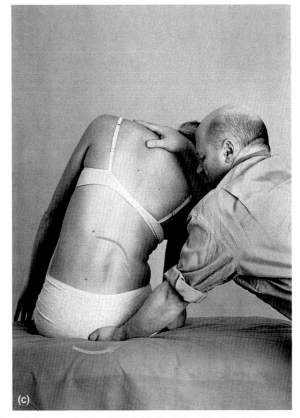

Figure 5.30 Examination of lateral fixation during lateral flexion of the torso to the right. (a) Lateral bend to the right shown on a skeleton, corresponding to phase 1. (b) Phase 1. (c) Phase 2.

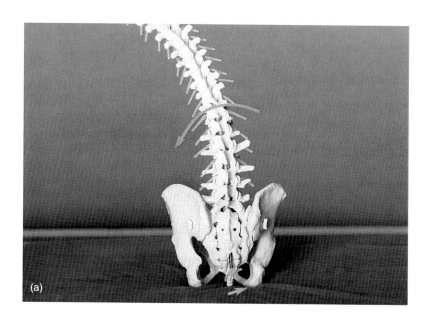

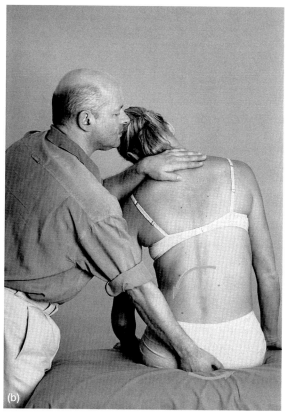

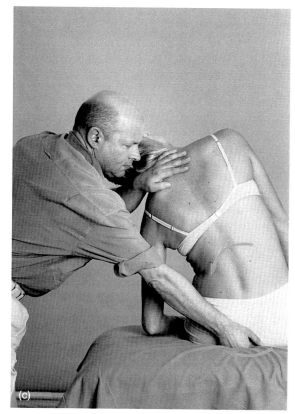

Figure 5.31   Examination of lateral fixation during lateral flexion of the torso to the left. (a) Lateral bend to the left shown on a skeleton, corresponding to phase 1. (b) Phase 1. (c) Phase 2.

Treatment techniques

Treatment of lateral fixation

Patient   Sitting on the treatment table, see above.

Therapist   Standing behind the patient, one knee bent on the table.

Contact   With the index and middle fingers on the side of the fixation between the coccyx and ischial tuberosity.

Action   The therapist positions the index and middle fingers on the fixated side laterally next to the coccyx and creates an elastic contact in the direction of the levator ani muscle and sacrotuberal ligament. The therapist compresses the patient's torso over the pectoral girdle and, in so doing, passively flexes the free side. The therapist's index and middle fingers remain in contact with the point of lateral fixation that was first touched (see above). The lateral flexion of the torso will push the coccyx farther into the fixation in the first phase. It is now important to maintain precise contact next to the coccyx and, in the case of a tangible change in tone, to apply a slight impulse in the cranial direction so as to slightly reinforce the lateral (and simultaneously anterior) displacement. At this moment, the therapist continues the lateral flexion of the torso. It should be kept in mind that this second phase of lateral flexion is not performed until the moment at which an actual change in tone can be felt on the fixated side of the coccyx. This change in tone can be exploited in order to guide the coccyx indirectly into motion toward the other side.

> This is a combined direct and indirect technique. We guide the coccyx farther into its fixation and thus indirectly achieve a release of the ligamentous structures. At the same time, we apply a direct impulse into the tone pattern of the levator ani muscle and directly stretch its fascial sheath by exerting pressure in the cranial direction in the pelvic floor. It is important to maintain the contact next to the coccyx in a precise manner. If the pressure acts directly on the coccyx, the anterior fixation may be reinforced.

Treatment of anterior fixation

Patient   Prone, legs extended, arms lying to the side next to the torso.

Therapist   Standing to the side at the level of the upper edge of the pelvis, facing in the distal direction.

Contact   With the index and middle fingers of one hand on the superficial posterior sacrococcygeal ligament and with the index and middle fingers of the other hand precisely below the coccyx.

Action   When the patient is prone, attention should be paid to the relative relaxation of the gluteal muscles. The therapist uses the index and middle fingers to create contact with the superficial posterior sacrococcygeal ligament. This contact should be elastic and, at the same time, achieve an intensity that transmits the contact into the periosteum of the last segment of the sacrum. With two fingers of the other hand, the therapist moves the coccyx slightly farther into its anterior fixation. The therapist now exerts intense, slowly sliding pressure on the fifth segment of the sacrum as if to release the fibers of the ligament from the periosteum located below it. The pressure should be applied along the individual arcs of the bone and not push the upper segments of the sacrum in the posterior direction.

> With some skill, it will be possible to indirectly loosen the sacrospinal ligament and, at the same time, reduce the strong tension on the posterior side of the sacrum that will have manifested as intraosseous tension in the case of long-ago injuries. The fingers on the coccyx follow with "listening"; the fingers on the posterior side of the sacrum exert active stretching force on connective tissue fibers and, at the same time, concentrate on "listening" to the bone structure located below the contact point.

After the mobilization of the sacrococcygeal joint, it is wise to examine the mobility of the sacrococcygeal joint again in the sitting position and, finally, to observe the mobility of the fifth segment of the sacrum supine.

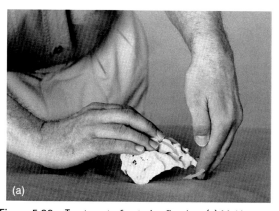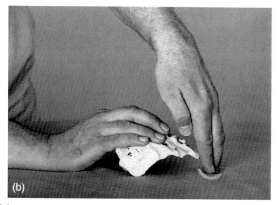

Figure 5.32   Treatment of anterior fixation. (a) Making contact. (b) Transmitting pressure.

If the injury to the joint was a very long time ago, then it is not only the fibers directly attached to the joint that are involved in the fixation. Over the course of time, the altered tensional pattern has also manifested in the sacroiliac ligament and the large-area fascial layers located above it such as the lumbar fascia.

In order to encourage a balanced tension between the deep ligament and tendon structures and the exterior sheath layers, it is advisable to use the following technique to act on the lumbar fascia and the tissue bed of the lumbar spine and the fascial layers adjacent to the lumbar area.

Treatment of fascial layers adjacent to the lumbar area

Patient   Supine, both legs extended, arms resting next to the torso.

Therapist   Standing to the side at the level of the thighs.

Contact   One hand holds the sacrum from the posterior direction while the other hand produces a contact with the lower third of the thoracolumbar fascia.

Action   It is important for this technique that the patient allows the weight of the pelvis and lower back to sink completely into the therapist's hands. The therapist supports the sacrum with one hand in such a way that the weight of the pelvis is evenly distributed. With the other hand, the therapist lifts the lower back region in a slight bend so that the muscle groups that run parallel to the spine relax slightly. Now, after the reduction in muscle tone, the relationship between the sacrum and the adjacent iliac bone and the lower lumbar vertebrae becomes tangible, particularly in the ligamentous bedding. While the therapist holds the lumbar spine area in a slight hyperlordosis, the therapist follows all movement of the sacrum that may occur, and finally applies a slight impulse in the region of the lower thoracolumbar fascia in the direction of the diaphragm and, at the same time, applies a gently pull to the lumbar fascia in the distal direction.

The precise mechanism of effect of this technique is described in the section regarding movement restrictions in the region of the lower lumbar spine (see section 4.1, Treatment of lumbar lordosis at the transition to the pelvic cavity and Treatment of flat back of the lumbar spine). Because the correction of the coccyx influences the tensional relationships in the spinal dura mater, it is advisable to subsequently examine the transition between the axis and foramen magnum. In practice, we frequently find compressions within the short section of the atlanto-occipital joint that disappear after the mobilization of the coccyx. However, the mobilization of the "lower pole" between the coccyx and sacrum can also cause an irritation at the transition of the upper pole between the atlas and base of the skull. For this reason, the connection between the upper cervical spine and head should be treated subsequently, if necessary.

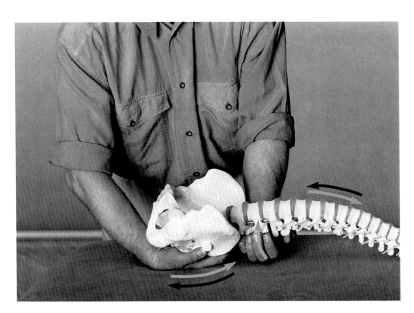

Figure 5.33   Treatment of fascial layers adjacent to the lumbar area.

5.4   JOINTS OF THE FOOT

As a rule, the transition between the foot and lower leg can be treated with techniques that have already been discussed in the section on the lower extremity (see section 4.5). However, there is a series of motion restrictions between the bones of the foot itself for which a special technique must be used that is applied directly to the joint surfaces. If movement restrictions have occurred in the bones of the foot, the self-regulation of the organism is subjected to certain limits by the structure of the arch of the foot. This is also the reason why the direct manipulation of these joints sometimes requires a considerable application of force and does not always meet with success.

If, for example, the navicular bone shows a limitation of motion in relation to the talus, if the cuboid bone shows a restriction of motion in relation to the calcaneus, or if a disruption of the spatial relationship occurs between the distal end of the tibia and the talus, the joint surfaces can quite literally lock into one another. The tendon and ligament structure of the arch of the foot, if it has a pronounced tension pattern, causes a long-lasting manifestation of this limitation of movement.

The following techniques take these facts into account. These are techniques that cause the major units of the foot to be distorted relative to one another such that the tensile forces of the plantar calcaneonavicular ligament and the long plantar ligament and the medial intermuscular septum are reduced during the application of the treatment technique. The relaxation of individual muscular insertions is secondary. The larger myofascial units of the foot are less important than the ligaments, particularly because the talus, which is so significant for the entire static situation of the foot and leg, does not serve as the origin or insertion of any muscle. In a manner of speaking, it is the keystone of the arch of the foot, whose relationships to the adjacent bones are dependent on the tensile force of the tendons and ligaments.

All of the mobilization techniques described here follow the same treatment strategy:

- The therapist gently exaggerates the relative spatial position of both foot bones to be mobilized, as is typical of the present fixation.

- At the same time, the therapist uses active pressure to distort the two bones relative to one another in such a way that they are somewhat released from the tension of the longitudinal arch of the foot caused by ligaments, tendons, and intermuscular septa and so that the surfaces of the joint can be moved.

If the techniques are applied successfully, the therapist's hands will feel a gradual scraping sound, although it cannot be heard by the human

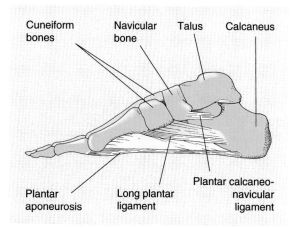

Cuneiform bones Navicular bone Talus Calcaneus

Plantar aponeurosis Long plantar ligament Plantar calcaneo-navicular ligament

Figure 5.34 Construction of the longitudinal arch of the foot from the medial direction.

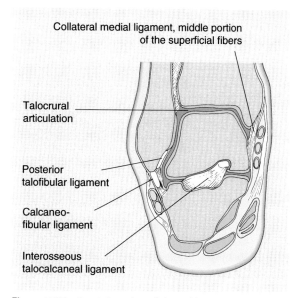

Collateral medial ligament, middle portion of the superficial fibers

Talocrural articulation

Posterior talofibular ligament

Calcaneo-fibular ligament

Interosseous talocalcaneal ligament

Figure 5.35 Frontal section of the ankle.

ear. This "sound" is caused by sliding of the compressed joint surfaces and can be interpreted as corresponding to the snap that occurs in direct joint manipulation.

Treatment of the joint between the talus and calcaneus

Patient Supine, one leg bent; the leg to be treated is extended.

Therapist Sitting at the foot.

Contact The therapist's thumb and front phalanges of one hand surround the calcaneus from the posterior side, while the therapist's other hand reaches in the direction of the talus on the medial collateral ligament.

Action Because the relationship between the talus and calcaneus is dependent upon the joint between the tibia and talus on the one side, and the distal end of the fibula and talus on the other side, it is important to observe the entire joint complex while applying the treatment technique. If the tibia appears to be displaced in the anterior direction on the talus, it is necessary to first manipulate this joint before we treat the subtle joint between the calcaneus and talus.

In order to mobilize the joint between the talus and calcaneus, the therapist's hands follow with "listening" until the end of the fixation tendency. In so doing, the therapist not only attempts to

focus his or her tactile senses on the two bones, but also observes the tensional forces originating from the interosseous talocalcaneal ligament. This ligament is positioned like a pillow between the two bones and has a great deal of significance in the stabilization and sliding ability of this joint.

As soon as the motion at the endpoint of the fixation has come to a standstill, the therapist distorts the talus and calcaneus more strongly relative to one another. The therapist holds the talus in its position and bends the calcaneus, which is easier to grasp, in the medial direction, as if it were a piece of mobile wood. At the same time, the therapist pushes the talus out of the fixation, using a very low level of subtle pressure of only a few grams. It is sometimes necessary to modify the direction in which the two bones are moved toward one another several times until the release of the fixation manifests, which occurs in minimal reverse movements.

Strictly speaking, this technique is a treatment of the ligamentous structures located laterally of the talus, i.e. the calcaneofibular ligament, which laterally connects the lower end of the fibula to the upper end of the calcaneus, and the calcaneotibial ligament, which medially connects the lower part of the tibia to the calcaneus. This technique influences the inner elasticity of the bone such that minimal changes in tension occur at points at which the tendons and ligaments are interconnected to the periosteum.

Treatment of the joint between the navicular bone and talus

Patient   Supine, one leg bent; the leg to be treated is extended.

Therapist   Sitting at the foot next to the treatment table.

Contact   With the fingers and thumbs of one hand on the navicular bone and the other hand on the talus.

Action   At this joint as well, the therapist uses both hands to follow with "listening" in order to sense the dominant direction in which the two bones want

to move closer to one another. If the navicular bone is displaced in the cranial direction, the cuneonavicular joint is affected as well. An increased tensile force of the long plantar ligament running between the cuneiform bones and an increase in tone of the posterior tibial muscle may be involved in the joint fixation between the navicular bone and the talus. In any event, it is advantageous in this situation to move the cuneiform bones and the talus toward one another so that the navicular bone slips farther in the cranial direction in its fixation and the long plantar ligament relaxes. It is not until this moment that the therapist begins to twist the navicular bone and talus toward each other, releases the cuneiform bones in the direction of the toes, and allows the navicular bone to follow the pull direction of the plantar calcaneonavicular ligament and glide out of the fixation.

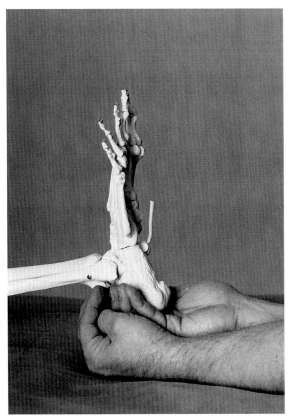

Figure 5.36   Treatment of the joint between the talus and calcaneus.

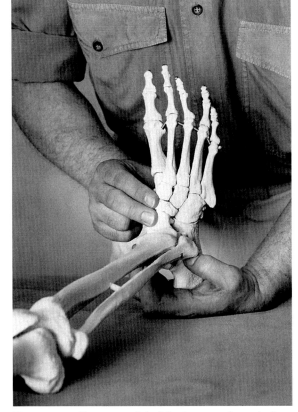

Figure 5.37   Treatment of the joint between the navicular bone and talus.

Treatment of the joints between the cuboid bone and calcaneus

Patient Supine, one leg bent; the leg to be treated is extended.

Therapist Sitting to the side at the foot.

Contact One palm supports the calcaneus from the medial direction and surrounds its exterior with the fingertips, while the other hand grasps the cuboid bone with the thumb and index finger.

Action While "listening," the therapist moves the calcaneus and the cuboid bone toward one another in such a way that, as in the previous techniques, the joint fixation becomes more pronounced. It should be borne in mind that, owing to the very individually pronounced shape of the foot, the directions in which we move the two bones together may vary greatly. As a rule, the bones also do not move in a linear fashion in their fixation, but rather on a tiny

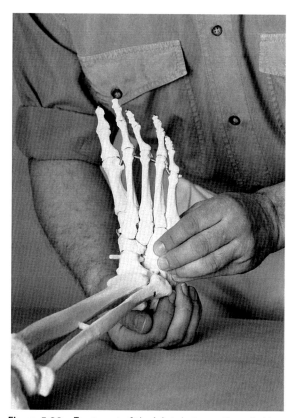

Figure 5.38 Treatment of the joints between the cuboid bone and calcaneus.

zigzag path. Because the cuboid bone, with its multiple joints with adjacent bones, has contact with various directional surfaces of the joint surface, it is very important to follow this zigzag path gradually until the endpoint of the joint fixation.

In this technique as well, the therapist uses a twisting of the arch of the foot in order to relax ligaments and aponeuroses in such a way that the restricted joint surfaces come into motion.

Treatment of intraosseous tension of the calcaneus

This technique is particularly suitable for treatment of healed fractures of the calcaneus.

Patient Supine, both legs extended, with the feet extending past the edge of the treatment table.

Therapist Sitting at the foot.

Contact With a relaxed palm on the calcaneus from the posterior direction, while the other hand supports the back of the hand.

Action The therapist takes the calcaneus with one palm in such a way that the hand precisely reflects the surface contour of the bone. While doing so, the therapist supports the back of the hand providing treatment with the palm of the other hand such that the patient's heel rests in both of the therapist's hands. The therapist first follows the calcaneus with "listening" into the position that the calcaneus wants to take in relation to the other adjacent bones and then allows this movement to come to its end. Sometimes the calcaneus will glide more strongly in the medial, lateral, anterior, or posterior direction. As a rule, this will not be a movement in a straight line, but rather more of an elliptical curve in which the calcaneus moves into the preferred position. Once it has arrived at the endpoint of this movement, the therapist reduces the intensity of the contact somewhat and now uses "listening" to first feel the periosteum of the calcaneus. The therapist now concentrates on whether individual points on the periosteum appear to be more compacted than others. At the same time, the therapist alters the quality of touch at these points as if to reach into the interior of the bone. This requires the therapist's palm to minimally compress the entire calcaneus, as if to squeeze out a sponge only a little. As soon as the counterforce coming from the interior of the bone intensifies against the compressing hand, the therapist reduces the compression, specifically in the directions in which the pressure from the interior of the bone is transmitted outward. This feels as if the bone were extending. Subsequently, the therapist's attention is again directed to the calcaneus in its relation to the adjacent bones and the calcaneus is allowed to slide back into its original position.

The treatment of intraosseous tension of the calcaneus greatly influences the joints of the ankle and metatarsus. I assume that the connection between the periosteum and adjacent tendons and ligaments is responsible for the efficacy of this technique. In the case of strongly pronounced muscle tone of the lower leg, I recommend a treatment variation: the therapist supports the calcaneus with only one hand and uses the other hand to support the lower leg from the posterior direction and performs the technique in this position.

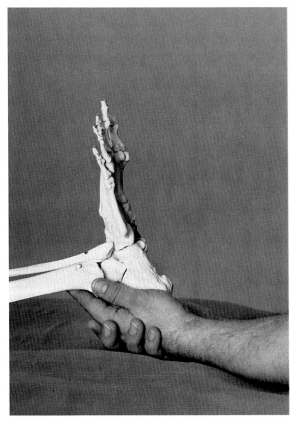

Figure 5.39 Hand position for treating intraosseous tension of the calcaneus.

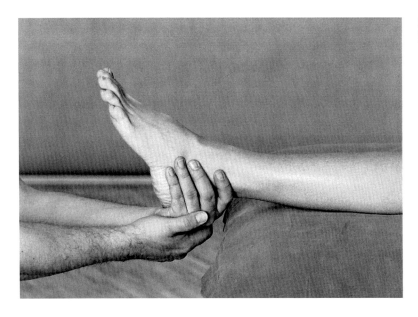

Figure 5.40 Treatment of intraosseous tension of the calcaneus.

Chapter 6

Visceral techniques in the myofascial context

From the traditional viewpoint of orthopedics and physical therapy, functional problems of the back and extremities are regarded as phenomena of the musculoskeletal system, and they are diagnosed and treated only in this context. This viewpoint experienced its first expansion when William Garner Sutherland applied the osteopathic concept to sutures of the cranium, the membranes of the craniosacral system, and the fluid systems associated with it. Sutherland's concepts have met with great interest today, in particular since John Upledger continued their use and development in his own craniosacral therapy. It was this craniosacral starting point that caused a shift in the way of thinking in the osteopathic discipline, which in the meantime had become focused only on joints, back to the aspect that the founder of the discipline, Andrew Taylor Still, had emphasized so greatly: the fasciae and membranes. To a certain extent, the craniosacral concept has led to a paradigm shift in osteopathy.

Similarly strong influences were felt at the beginning of the 1980s, when the concept of visceral manipulation was published for the first time. Barral and Mercier presented a diagnosis and treatment concept which, for the first time, made the visceral organs a systematically described part of manual treatment strategy. At the beginning, emphasis was not placed on the organs, but rather on investigating their context in the musculoskeletal system. During his clinical practice, Barral had the opportunity of investigating specific diseases (primarily severe diseases of the lungs), as well as their effects on the spine, in greater detail and later on, after the demise of the patient, comparing the results of the examination with the autopsy findings. In so doing, he came across a groundbreaking observation: if it was possible to detect tuberculous caverns on one side of the lung, considerable changes were found in autopsy in the region of the cervical spine. Barral placed these changes in relation to the restrictions of movement that he had been able to ascertain as a tactile finding while the patient was alive.

As early as the beginning of the 1970s, Barral used this observation as a starting point for extensive practical research, which resulted in an extremely differentiated treatment concept. Beginning from the first edition of *Visceral Manipulation*, which came out in 1983, he has constantly been elaborating, testing, and refining this concept in practical and technical terms.

Mobility and motility of organs

The treatment goal of "mobilization" did not included only the musculoskeletal elements of the organism; it was also extended to the relational movement of organs. In a certain sense, this allowed the organs to be assigned as if they formed "joints" by way of their sheaths of connective tissue and ligamentous connections, and these "joints" displayed regular and irregular movement behavior comparable to a joint of the musculoskeletal system.

In the section covering treatment of the breathing pattern (see section 4.1, Tests to evaluate breathing movement), we were able to see that the "joint movement" of the organs is passive motion caused by movement of the diaphragm. Axes of movement that are characteristic for an organ and spatial curves that are related to the visceral cavity and neighboring organs can be described. The existence of these axes of movement and spatial curves may be plausibly reconstructed by considering the organ cavities and ligaments of the organs, as well as the existing sliding layer, a "special form of fluid connective tissue." Ultimately, regular motion and deviations of motion can be examined with reproducible manual tests.

In addition to organ motion caused by breathing, i.e. mobility, which is easily acceptable from

a traditional viewpoint, Barral also described an active movement originating from the inner dynamics from the organs themselves. He called this subtle form of movement, which can be discerned only with the greatest sensitivity, "motility" (Barral and Mercier 2002: 8).

Motility consists of two phases:

- a movement phase, which Barral refers to as "expir," moves the organ closer to the central axis of the body
- the countermovement, "inspir," moves the organ away from the central axis.

One characteristic of this movement, the motility of the organs, is that a synchronous rhythm manifests in all of the organs. Peculiarly, there is no direct correlation between mobility, which is caused by breathing, and the subtle movement of motility with regard to the directions of motion. In some organs, there are overlapping movements, and in others mobility and motility are completely different.

Barral explains the phenomenon of motility as follows: he attributes this form of movement to the axis rotations that individual organs make during embryonic development. With the aid of this embryological model, Barral interprets the motility of the organs as a lasting trace of movement from embryonic development. Thus, motility would be a subtle pendulum movement between the actual position of the organ and the spatial curve that led to this position during embryonic development. In a manner of speaking, motility is a sort of "movement memory" of the organs.

Barral also developed a manual, axis-oriented diagnostic pattern for this form of organ movement, i.e. motility, which allows us to evaluate regular movements and deviations in a manual diagnostic manner.

Beyond manual diagnostics, however, it has been difficult up to now to objectify motility. It would be very difficult to develop an empirical method of measurement that would be able to register the motility of the organs. However, there are sufficient signs in practice that show us that motility is a phenomenon of movement whose treatment allows us to attain remarkable results. In my opinion, these results are remarkable primarily because they do not only influence motility itself, but rather their effects manifest in the area of phenomena of joint function and segmental alignment of sections of the body, which is far easier to grasp.

Therefore, the assumption is obvious that the more refined motility, in addition to the substantially more massive mobility, has an influence on the interior dynamics of the visceral cavities and is a factor of form adaptation, which is present in all processes of life.

I assume that mobility and motility of organs are initially reflected in the membranous inner construction of visceral cavities. I also assume that the dynamics of the organs are an influencing factor on the exterior parietal structure of the torso and ultimately have an effect into the fascia (see Rolf 1993: 140).

Consequences for treatment

For the practice of fascial and membrane techniques, this assumption has the consequence that, in treatment techniques that are aimed at stabilization of form, we must take into account the mobility and motility of organs. In treatment practice, therefore, we must examine the organs in a detailed manner and only then can we classify our findings in a larger form and movement context.

To repeat our central hypothesis, the connective tissue sheaths of the organs also form a network of bridges between musculoskeletal, nervous, and visceral components. For this reason, treatment of a fixation that has been diagnosed as visceral is not only treatment of the fixation itself, but also at the same time a treatment of all fascial layers formed and maintained by repetitive movement patterns that are connected to the organ or even only spatially assigned to it.

The following techniques must be understood in this context. Based on Barral's concept of organ mobilization, I have attempted to develop a treatment strategy by means of which individual elements of the visceral system are mobilized in the context of form of the walls and intermediate layers of the parietal structure of the visceral system. In my opinion, we can derive treatment steps from this that, for example, increase the motility of the lungs in that they simultaneously improve the inner form of the chest cavity and the exterior capacity for movement associated with it. Or the movement capacity, the mobility of the liver and diaphragm,

can be influenced in such a way that influence is exerted at the same time on the intercostal membranes and thus an improvement of function in the costovertebral joints is achieved. The goal of these techniques is to simultaneously regulate the equilibrium of movement of parts of the organism as well as the stability of the whole.[1]

Treatment of the mobility of the liver according to Barral

Patient   Sitting on a bench.

Therapist   Standing behind the patient.

Contact   With the gently applied outer edges of both hands (without the fingertips) slightly below the lower boundary of the liver.

Action   The therapist guides both hands below the right costal arch while the patient slouches slightly in order to relax the abdominal musculature. If the liver tends to be fixated in the pattern of inhalation, i.e. sinks more prominently in the direction of the navel, in this body position its right section will be clearly tangible on the therapist's hands. Because the liver and diaphragm are lower when sitting than when lying down, this tendency appears to be reinforced in the inferior direction. The therapist is now able to lift the liver against the diaphragm in the anterior direction in the manner described by Barral and thus sometimes achieves a redistribution of the serosal layer between Glisson's capsule and the adjacent organs. However, the therapist can also maintain elastic contact with the organ without changing its position, guide the patient into more of a slouched posture and then guide the patient back into a straighter posture. This allows the therapist to achieve a displacement of the entire peritoneal space relative to the adjacent diaphragm. The therapist can now ensure that this displacement manifests at the lowest sections of the boundary surface between the peritoneum and diaphragm. Thus, the therapist can gently rotate the upper body relative to the abdominal cavity while the therapist's hands constantly maintain the contact below the liver and affect the ligamentous suspension of the organ. Here, it is important that the quality of the touch be

---

[1] A summary of the anatomy relevant for visceral treatment can be found in Barral and Mercier (2002).

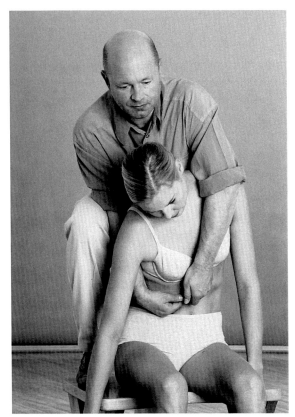

Figure 6.1   Treatment of the mobility of the liver according to Barral.

constantly supportive and that any drastic impulse against the organ be avoided.

> In cases in which the movement of the entire liver is limited by a stricture of its sheath layer, for example, it is recommended that the therapist support the primary part of the organ from the right with only one hand and use the other hand to contact the narrowly pronounced left portion of the liver. In this case as well, mobilization happens by turning and tilting the lower part of the chest in relation to the abdomen while the liver is supported.

Treatment of the motility of the liver in the case of an inspir fixation

For this technique, it is essential to bear in mind that the so-called inspir movement of the liver, its

motility, occurs spatially in countermotion to the mobility, i.e. breathing movement. The therapist should therefore pay no attention to inhalation and exhalation that are caused by the motion of the diaphragm.

Patient   Lying on the right side, both knees bent.

Therapist   Standing at the level of the hips.

Contact   The patient lies with the right side of the lower chest cavity, i.e. the exterior structure of the hepatic cavity, precisely on the therapist's right palm; at the same time the therapist uses the other hand to create contact with the lower left half of the thorax.

Action   The therapist's tactile senses are directed exclusively at the subtle motility of the organ. This process is facilitated by the fact that the patient is resting with a fully relaxed side on the therapist's hand and the therapist is surrounding the structure of the ribcage in such a way as to be able to feel through it and sense the subtle movement of the liver. The inspir movement of the organ manifests as a rotation in the posterior–superior direction. If this movement is dominant, i.e. if the liver is fixated in the inspir movement, the therapist's hand will receive the impression that the liver tends to press against the posterior–superior section of the space below the diaphragm. It appears to have more weight at the top and back and the rotational expir movement is only dimly implied. Under no circumstances should the therapist force the organ into the limited expir movement. Rather, the therapist exerts a subtle compression on the thoracic wall surrounding the liver, as if to slightly compress the frame of a drum, and allows the tendencies of the liver to sink farther into the inspir fixation. This process can be facilitated using the other hand in the region of the lower left chest cavity by supporting the same inspir motion of the stomach. This should guide the stomach into a reinforced inspir movement in turn only if its own motility capacity allows it to do so.

The efficacy of this technique is primarily based on the fact that a liver caught in the inspir movement is automatically lowered somewhat in the direction of the fixation by the position of the body and, at the same time, the therapist contributes to a relaxation of the exterior sheath structure.

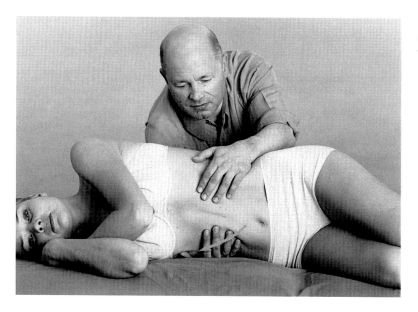

Figure 6.2   Treatment of the motility of the liver in the case of an inspir fixation.

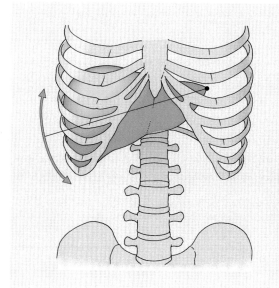

Figure 6.3   Motility of the liver in the frontal plane according to Barral.

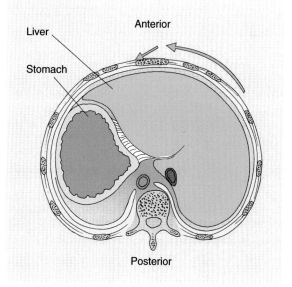

Figure 6.4   Motility of the liver in the horizontal plane according to Barral.

In applying this technique, it is essential that the therapist knows the axis of motility precisely and compares the amplitude of inspir and expir. As in the induction techniques described by Jean-Pierre Barral, it is important to clearly recognize the movement that describes a larger spatial curve.

The goal is therefore to reinforce the motility movement with the larger range of motion until the countermovement manifests more clearly. Barral emphasized that, even in the case of unlimited motility, i.e. when there is no fixation in the inspir or expir, it can be advisable to apply the induction principle. In addition, he emphasized that, in this

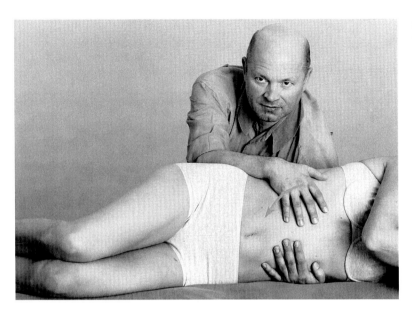

Figure 6.5 Treatment of expir fixation of the liver.

process, the motility of an organ can temporarily come to a standstill.[2]

Treatment of expir fixation of the liver

Patient Lying on the left side, knees slightly bent.

Therapist Standing at the level of the hips.

Contact This time, the patient lies with the side of the stomach on the therapist's left hand. The therapist's other hand touches the area of the lower right chest cavity.

Action The therapist's left hand supports the left chest cavity in the area of the boundary between the stomach and diaphragm subtly enough to be able to observe the motility of the stomach. At the same time, the therapist's other hand feels the motility of the liver in the area of the lower right chest cavity. If an expir fixation is present, i.e. if the motility is more intensified in the anterior and inferior directions, this is reinforced by the patient lying on one side, particularly if the patient's body is tilted

[2] "If a standstill of movement occurs during visceral induction, it is best to wait ten to twenty seconds and then carefully initiate the movement again, initially in the direction that displayed the lowest degree of resistance to movement before induction. If the therapist has done this correctly, the visceral motility returns within one minute, intensified and in the normal direction of movement." (Barral and Mercier 2002: 23)

ever so slightly in the anterior direction. The therapist now uses the push of the peritoneal space in the anterior and superior directions and supports the expir movement of the liver simultaneously with the expir movement of the stomach. In this case as well, influence should be exerted on the motility of the stomach only if it is free. As soon as a countermovement begins to make itself felt, the therapist supports it in a very subtle fashion, as if to follow the movement of a pendulum. If no "rest point" is established, it is advisable to guide both organs through the movement cycle several times.

Treatment of the motility of the lungs

Patient In the dorsal position, both legs extended.

Therapist Sitting to the side at the level of the chest cavity.

Contact Both hands precisely under the axis of movement of one lung, the little finger side of both hands on the treatment table.

Action The therapist produces supportive contact with the upper chest cavity in such a way that it imitates the dominant shape of the curvature of the inner wall of the chest. In so doing, the surface of each of the therapist's index fingers traces precisely the course of the vertical and diagonal axis of movement of one lung.

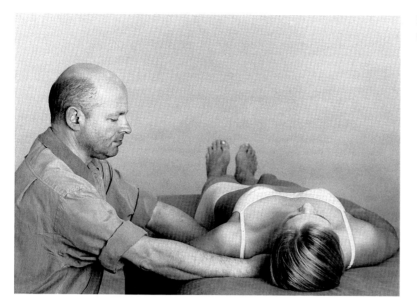

Figure 6.6   Treatment of the motility of the lungs.

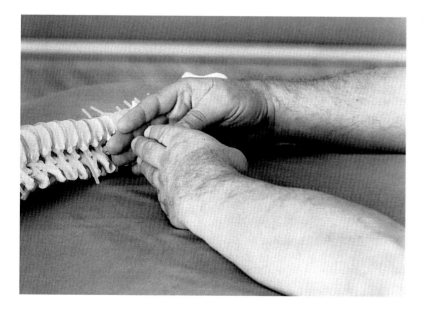

Figure 6.7   Hand position.

The therapist first observes the motility of the lungs. If a dominant direction of movement is evident, then the therapist intensifies it. This means that the expir movement is intensified if it is dominant. However, if the inspir movement is more strongly tangible, it is supported correspondingly. Because the lungs themselves can only follow the movements of their walls, we must rely on tracing the dominant motility in the intermediate layers of the chest cavity. In other words, we push the parietal pleura in the direction of the dominant motility and support this movement additionally by an extremely careful compression of the costal–muscular–membrane structure of the exterior chest cavity. Then we reduce this compression so that the development of the motility in the limited direction is facilitated.

The objective of our global treatment is to reduce or even eliminate detail fixations while we include the inner form in which these fixations have left their mark.

The motility of the lungs can be felt only if the musculature of the back is completely relaxed. Because motility and mobility have identical axes in the region of the lungs, it is possible to practice this technique using the mobility motion, which is far easier to feel. The initial goal is to feel the inner rotational movement of the lungs along their axes.

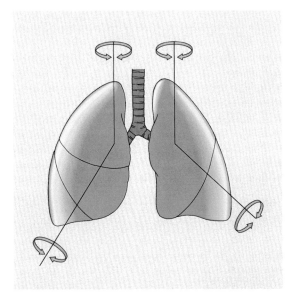

Figure 6.8 Mobility and motility of the lungs (according to Barral).

After the treatment of one side of the lungs, it is always advisable to examine the other side of the lungs and, if necessary, perform the treatment described above in an analogous manner. Subsequently, it should be possible to harmonize the oscillating movement of both lungs between a posterior position and an anterior position. For this purpose, the therapist places one hand under the space of each lung from the posterior direction and supports the exterior arch of the back along the part of the axis of movement of the lungs that runs diagonally outward until comparable amplitudes of movement have been established on both sides.

Treatment of the mobility of the kidney in relation to the psoas muscle

Patient   Prone.

Therapist   Sitting at the level of the hips.

Contact   Between the duodenum and colon just below the kidney while the other hand supports the thigh on the half of the body being treated.

Action   The therapist first produces a gentle contact on the abdominal wall, then gradually uses the ball of the thumb to reach between the duodenum and colon until it is possible to transmit the effect of the contact in the direction of the retroperitoneal space. Because the lower boundary of a healthy kidney cannot be felt, it is advisable to produce the

Figure 6.9   Treatment of the mobility of the kidney in relation to the psoas muscle.

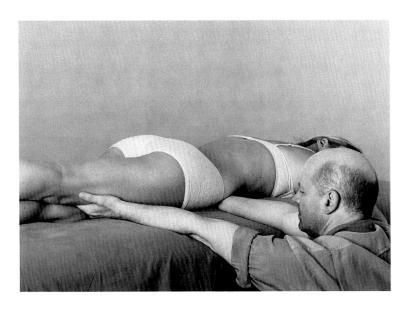

contact somewhat below the normal position instead. In the case of a normally mobile kidney, the therapist will feel a slight but clearly tangible push against the hand. This push will not occur in the case of a fixation of the kidney, nor will it occur in the case of a sinking of the kidneys. The therapist's other hand now supports the patient's leg on the side of the kidney to be treated on the other leg so that the ankles are resting on one another. The inner rotation occurring on the leg causes a slight extension of the psoas muscle that is sufficient to increase somewhat the scope of movement available to the adjacent kidney. Now, every time the patient exhales, the therapist applies a minimal push laterally of the psoas in the cranial direction and slightly in the medial direction, i.e. diagonally relative to the center line of the organism. In so doing, the therapist avoids any direct mechanical push against the kidney. Rather, the therapist's goal is a gentle movement impulse in the retroperitoneal section that is available to the kidney as its range of movement.

Stabilization of the peritoneal cavity relative to the retroperitoneal and subperitoneal cavity

Patient   Prone.

Therapist   Sitting at the level of the abdominal cavity.

Contact   With the palm of one hand providing support in the lower region of the sternum and the adjacent ribs; the other hand below the navel in the region of the small intestine.

Action   The therapist uses one hand to support the lower chest cavity while the other hand accepts the lower peritoneal cavity as if the organs were sinking more and more into this hand. Using the hand placed on the lower chest cavity, the therapist tries to make contact with the lowest portion of the retrosternal transversus thoracis and its fascia as well as the uppermost part of the transversus abdominis and its fascia. The fibers of the uppermost part of the transversus abdominis and the lowest part of the transversus thoracis have the same orientation in this section.

The therapist now moves the fingers and heel of the supporting hand more closely together so that the flexion movement of the two muscles is supported, and, at the same time, pushes the fingers and heel of that hand in the cranial direction in order to achieve an effect transverse to the direction of the fascial fibers. Thus, the therapist lifts the chest cavity slightly. At the same time, the therapist uses the other hand to follow any rotational movements that occur if they manifest in a two-dimensional fashion in the peritoneum or in a counter-clockwise direction. If these movements occur, the therapist intensifies them and then waits

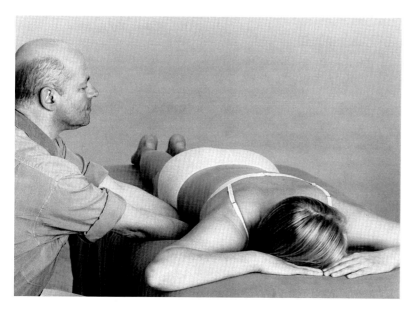

Figure 6.10   Stabilization of the peritoneal cavity relative to the retroperitoneal and subperitoneal cavity.

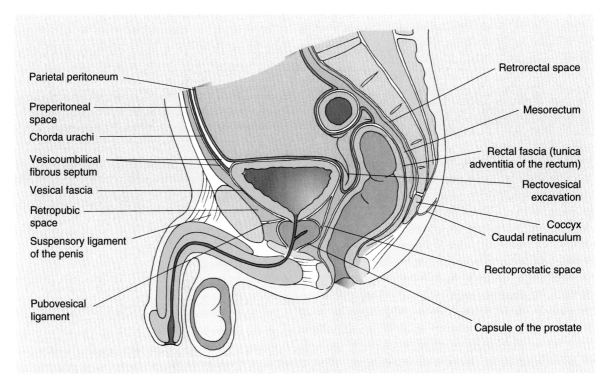

Figure 6.11   Medial section of the pelvis of the male to show the connective tissue cavities.

Parietal peritoneum

Preperitoneal space

Chorda urachi

Vesicoumbilical fibrous septum

Vesical fascia

Retropubic space

Suspensory ligament of the penis

Pubovesical ligament

Retrorectal space

Mesorectum

Rectal fascia (tunica adventitia of the rectum)

Rectovesical excavation

Coccyx
Caudal retinaculum

Rectoprostatic space

Capsule of the prostate

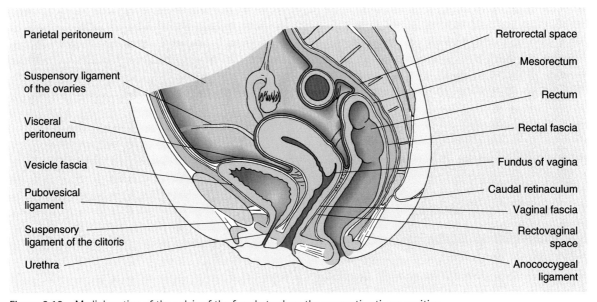

Figure 6.12   Medial section of the pelvis of the female to show the connective tissue cavities.

Parietal peritoneum

Suspensory ligament of the ovaries

Visceral peritoneum

Vesicle fascia

Pubovesical ligament

Suspensory ligament of the clitoris

Urethra

Retrorectal space

Mesorectum

Rectum

Rectal fascia

Fundus of vagina

Caudal retinaculum

Vaginal fascia

Rectovaginal space

Anococcygeal ligament

until a countermovement occurs and then follows this movement to a resting point. While the contact is maintained unabated in the region of the lower chest cavity, the therapist now uses the hand placed on the lower chest cavity to push the peritoneum and the organs it contains in a sliding manner relative to the retroperitoneal cavity. While doing so, the therapist uses "listening" as well.

Because this technique can affect the connection and possible adhesions between the posterior layer of the peritoneum and fascia of the kidney, any mechanical jerking or stretching should be avoided. Rather, the contact should act layer by layer through the peritoneum into the retroperitoneal cavity such that a somewhat "inductive" stretching occurs in the connective tissue bedding of the organs at points where the density of the tissue has increased.

> This technique may be varied in order to treat the relationship between the subperitoneal and peritoneal cavities in that the therapist selects a contact point farther below directly transverse of the pubic bone rather than in the lower abdominal cavity and, in so doing, touches the ligamentous connection between the bladder and pubic bone. In the case of a bladder fixation, the therapist now keeps this contact point and, with the other hand, switches from the lower chest cavity to the lower abdominal cavity. With this hand, the therapist moves the entire complex of the small intestine toward the bladder in such a way that the pressure from the bladder is transmitted onto the pubic bone. In the male, care must be taken that the hand on the pubic bone does not exert any acute contact on the spermatic ducts; in the woman, caution is advisable in the region of the ovaries, which cannot be felt. In a second step, the therapist moves the lower peritoneal cavity with its organs in the anterocranial direction while the other hand supports the ligamentous connection between the bladder and pubic bone just above the pubic bone.

Summarizing aspects

At the beginning of this chapter, I made reference to the fact that Barral has described axes of mobility and motility for all organs. In the light of the central hypothesis that it is the fascial and membrane system that reacts to increased pressure and tension conditions with changes in fiber density, fiber orientation, and fluid balance, organ movements can be understood as the motor of inner form. If, for example, the connective tissue sheath of an organ is reacting to a chronic inflammation, changes occur in the venous return flow from the organ as well as to the gas or fluid status of a hollow organ. Moreover, along with the axis of movement of the organ, the orientation of the organ column in the entire space of the torso changes as well. This change to the inner form also forces the exterior myofascial system into different tension patterns. Thus, it becomes comprehensible why a restriction of movement of a kidney on one side leads to one side of the torso being slouched from inside and compensatory changes occur in the region of the neck.

In general, we can say that changes in the retroperitoneal cavity have a direct effect on the prevertebral area. Thus, influence may be felt on one section of the curvature of the spine which as a result can be transmitted to all other spinal curvatures. So it is possible that, as a result of a fixation of the left kidney caused by impact from a traffic accident, for example, the form of the curvature of the spine could change at the transition between the lumbar and thoracic spine. Without pain necessarily occurring in this area itself, compensatory reactions occur farther in the cranial direction, in the region of the cervical spine, which then cause chronic discomfort on the left side as well and cannot be cured in the long term by local treatment of the neck.

It is not easy to produce a simple schema to explain the effect of organ fixations on the curvatures of the spine and the general segmented posture of the organism. However, we can name fundamental tendencies that we encounter again and again in practice. Thus, we can establish that there is a close connection in the lower pelvic region between the sacrum and the organs of the pelvis. Organ fixations in this region change the tilt angle of this section of the body in the sense of a greater tilt in the anterior or posterior direction. They can also influence the tendency of both alae of the ilium to move more strongly into the inflare or outflare position.

As we have already seen in the chapter on breathing (Chapter 4), the organs located directly below the diaphragm influence the excursion space of the diaphragm. As a result, we primarily encounter changes in the transitional passages between the chest cavity and shoulders. Changes to organs in the chest cavity itself, to the fascial–ligamentous bridge between the upper cupulas of the pleura and the neck, lead to lasting changes in the region of the cervical spine.

It is certainly not possible to explain the relationships behind these form and movement events entirely with changes in direction of shear and pull forces alone. We should assume that the entire nerve supply of various elements of the body plays a role as well. A typical example is the role that the phrenic nerve must play simultaneously in the region of the shoulder and the triangular ligaments of the liver.[3]

---

[3] I refer here to the section performed by Professor Arnaud and Jean-Pierre Barral in 1972 (Hôpital de la Tronche, Grenoble).

Chapter 7

Treatment of the mandibular joint and the craniosacral system

There is probably no field within the manual discipline that is as controversial as the craniosacral system. There are a number of reasons for this:

- Within its shell of vertebrae and cranial bones, the craniosacral system cannot be perceived using common diagnostic techniques.
- The palpation of mobility and restrictions of motion in the craniosacral system requires an extraordinary level of sensitivity and patience on the part of the therapist.
- The scope of movement that is present at the joints between the bones is so small that its palpability is constantly being placed in question by mainstream medicine.
- The options for explaining the fluctuations in pressure that are described as rhythmic are difficult to understand.[1]

It certainly did not facilitate an unbiased discussion of the craniosacral concept that some advocates of the discipline described it in a mystical style with religious overtones. The issue of whether the founder of the method, William G. Sutherland, supported this sort of development with certain aspects of his basic approach is perhaps no longer very significant today. In any event, a documentation of the original concept can be found in notes

---

[1] See the critical and extraordinarily perceptive description by A. Abehsera (2000 and 2002).

from his course published by Anne L. Wales that deserves to be taken seriously even by the skeptics (Sutherland 1990: 281–2).

Interestingly, there are no references in these class notes to the idea that the craniosacral system should be treated in isolation from the other systems of the organism. In a surprisingly direct manner, it clearly refers to the restrictions of the musculoskeletal and visceral systems. For both fields, the documentation shows a series of manipulations that are illustrated with photographs and make clear that Sutherland advocated a very broad basic approach in his treatment practice.

It is also this aspect that justifies my opinion that the craniosacral system should first be examined independently of the model of the craniosacral pulse. The techniques for treatment of the mandibular joint described below represent an effort in this direction. In a certain way, these techniques take into account the traditional concept of flexion and extension of the craniosacral system; however, there are fundamental differences in the practical procedures in comparison with the classical craniosacral approach.

I assume that the components of the craniosacral system are connected to the universal fascial and membrane connections in the same manner as all types of tissue. It is certain that the relative isolation in a partially closed system causes a certain independent dynamic. In practice, we encounter constellations again and again in which the problem has manifested primarily within the craniosacral context and which also appear to be treatable only within that context. However, there are numerous other connections: craniosacral tension patterns and restrictions of movement often have an effect on the myofascial system of the large visceral cavities, the interior of the ribcage, the abdominal cavity, and the pelvic cavity. Because the fasciae and membranes function like locks in the access passages of the fluid systems, they influence the intracranial pressure and therefore the intracranial membrane system as well. Even muscle tone plays a role at the transitions of the cranium and between the lumbar spine and sacrum. Finally, there is also one other direct connection to the spinal dura mater from the vertebral canal into the fascial layers of the musculature by way of the direct connection to the perineurial sheaths.

My hypothesis is that, in various respects, the independent dynamic of the craniosacral system is able to develop as a micromovement only as far as the membranes in the region of the adjacent sections of the body allow it to do so. The tension of the intracranial membranes is extensively dependent on the pressure of bodily fluids that arrive in the interior of the cranium by way of the neck and flow back out by way of the neck into the chest cavity. In order to be able to maintain an intracranial equilibrium of the membranes, unrestricted inward and outward flows are necessary. I think that, to a certain degree, the complexity of the craniosacral system can be circumvented if, in the course of our treatment, we first concentrate on freeing the inward and outward paths of restrictions. Thus, the craniosacral system has the ability to regulate itself to a large extent. Only after this step is it possible that a detailed craniosacral correction in the original sense may be necessary.

Moreover, there is yet another aspect that suggests an "extracranial" treatment strategy for the cranium: the cranium is in a myofascial, ligamentous, and membranous connection to the mandible. In many patients, it is precisely in this one connection where the center of tension of the entire organism may be found. Presumably, this connection plays a central role in the craniosacral system in areas other than dysfunction of the mandibular joint as well.

The connection between the cranium and the mandible is subjected to a constant dynamic during speaking and swallowing as well as to considerable fluctuations in pressure during chewing. The pressure acts on layers that are connected to a highly sensitive control system by way of masticatory surfaces. It is thus possible for us to sense even minimal discrepancies of fractions of a millimeter on masticatory surfaces.

In this chapter, a number of techniques are introduced that are particularly suitable for treating dysfunction of the mandibular joint. If they are applied to transitions from the chest cavity to the neck and the neck to the head, they are also suitable, independently of mandibular joint dysfunction, for the treatment of cranial tension patterns in the intracranial region of both membranes and sutures.

Anatomy of the fasciae

The mandibular joint is at particular risk of being influenced by an increase in the tone of the musculature as well as by tension forces from other regions of the body transmitted by the connections of the fascial system. At the same time, it is constantly subjected to varying pressures due to its role in the act of swallowing. In a certain sense, the mandibular joint can be described as the buffer zone for opposing force vectors. Immense pressures can act on the mandibular joint if the tone pattern of the muscles that run between the upper and lower jaw is elevated. In such a situation, the mandible is constantly being pushed against the maxilla while, at the same time, tension forces are acting in the opposite direction, i.e. in the inferior direction toward the neck and chest cavity. The fine structure of the mandibular joint itself is able only up to a certain point to cushion the combination of pull and shear forces that occur in this process.

The fasciae of the neck region play an important role in the transmission of these active forces. Anatomy differentiates between three fascial layers in the region of the neck:

- a superficial layer, the superficial lamina of the cervical fasciae
- a middle layer, the pretracheal lamina of the cervical fasciae
- a deep layer, the prevertebral lamina of the cervical fasciae.

It is a peculiarity of the superficial fascia lamina of the neck that it is located not only under the skin, but also under the platysma. Below the platysma, this layer forms a direct connection from the mandible and clavicles to the sternum. The connection to the sternum in the inferior direction plays a particularly important role because the superficial lamina ends at this point and does not extend any farther over the surface of the sternum. At individual points, this superficial layer has a connection to the deeper, middle-layer fascia of the neck and connects to the hyoid bone and its greater horn. In the posterior region, it is connected to the highly elastic layers of the nuchal ligament and it surrounds the trapezius muscles.

The middle fascia of the neck, which runs farther inward, is less laminar than the exterior layer.

It extends from the hyoid bone in the inferior direction down to the interior surface of the clavicles and sternum. In contrast to the exterior layer, it is in close connection with the visceral components of the neck that have a longitudinal path: the trachea, the esophagus, and also the thyroid gland and larynx. It is also connected to the next deepest fascial layer, the prevertebral fascia, specifically at the level of the thyroid gland. At both lateral edges, it adheres to the fascial sheath of the sternocleidomastoid muscle.

The deepest layer of the fascia of the neck, the prevertebral lamina of the cervical fasciae, plays the most significant role for the techniques. I describe for treating the transitions between the chest cavity, neck, and cranium: it is connected at the same time to elements of the deep structure and superficial structure and is part of the fascial sheath of the prevertebral muscles of the neck, i.e. the longus coli, the rectus capitis anterior, and the longus capitis. To the side of the neck, it comes into a connection with the longitudinal vessels and, in the anterior direction, it is loosely connected to the sliding layer of the retropharyngeal connective tissue. It also has connections to the levator scapulae and, in its posterior region, to the superficial fascia (Waldeyer 1993: 152).

For the transition between the upper chest cavity and the lower neck cavity it is significant because it is connected to the endothoracic fascia, which in turn is connected to the peritoneum in the nearest transitional area in the inferior direction. The thoracic fascia there forms the bridge between the inner sheath layer of both large visceral cavities and the prevertebral layers of the neck. In the cranial direction, there is finally one other connection of the deep fascia of the neck with the pharyngobasilar fascia and thus to the nasopharyngeal space.[2]

In the context of the cervical fasciae, the nuchal ligament is also significant because it also has an important bridging function between the superficial and deep layers: on the one hand, coming from the deep layers of the occiput, it is connected to all posterior processes of the cervical spine, but it also has a large-surface insertion in the fascia of

---

[2] See the description of the nasopharyngeal space in Liem (2000: 415–23).

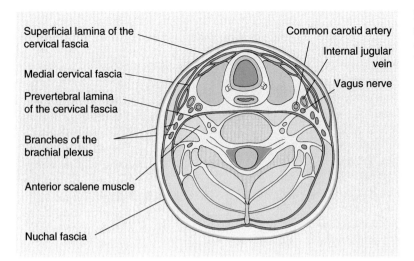

Superficial lamina of the cervical fascia

Medial cervical fascia

Prevertebral lamina of the cervical fascia

Branches of the brachial plexus

Anterior scalene muscle

Nuchal fascia

Common carotid artery

Internal jugular vein

Vagus nerve

Figure 7.1 Cross-section of the neck at the level of the first tracheal cartilage: course of the cervical fasciae.

the trapezius muscle in the upper region of the chest cavity.

The superficial fascia of the neck ends on the clavicles and, in the inferior direction, it is connected to the fascial layers of the thoracic musculature. In the cranial direction, it meets the lower boundary of the fascia of the masticatory musculature on the mandible. An important fascial layer for our treatment techniques in this area is the temporal fascia, which extends as a large plate of connective tissue between the superior temporal line and the zygomatic arch. The fascial sheaths of the smaller masticatory muscles are of secondary significance. Finally, the pterygotemporomandibular aponeurosis plays an important role in the techniques described below for correction of the lateral deviation of the mandible when opening the mouth.[3]

Notes on diagnostics

In view of the complex structure of the mandibular joint and its many connections in the region of the head and neck, it stands to reason that we should ensure our diagnosis by examining its relationship to the masticatory surfaces. Unfortunately, in recent years, it has not been possible to confirm

long-postulated connections between tooth status and surface morphology of the mandibular joint.[4]

As reasonable and necessary as corrections to bite surfaces may be, their positive effect appears to primarily lie in a better distribution of pressure on the teeth, but not in the region of the mandibular joint.

The diagnostic situation is complicated by the fact that the imaging techniques cannot fulfill the expectations that were initially placed on them. The articular disk, which plays such an important role in normal joint function, is shown on MRI images as a structure rich in collagen fibers, a low-signal zone (Müller 1990: 138).

As Müller has convincingly described, it is sometimes possible to confuse the disk with other low-signal structures because imaging methods do not allow a clear distinction between ligamentous and tendon elements and hard tissue structures on the one hand and the disk on the other hand. Unfortunately, the diagnostic value of endoscopy appears to be very limited in the region of this joint as well (Müller 1990: 141).

The examination of the active and passive movement sequence at the mandibular joint is initially sufficient for a manual diagnosis. If there is suspicion of morphological changes, the diagnostic

---

[3] See the description in Liem (2000: 270) (in reference to Perlemuter and Waligora).

[4] Müller (1990: 129–30) assumes that there is no simple or strict correlation between the biomechanical facts of the masticatory system and joint morphology.

advice of a dentist is indispensable. The important question here is that of etiology and the concrete manifestation of the morphological changes. Müller made groundbreaking observations with regard to a typology in his research on autopsy preparations. Apparently the limited sliding ability of the articular disk primarily arises in the context of two circumstances: either pronounced osseous changes in shape are present on the surface of the fossa or surface changes in the form of "roughness" occur on the cranial edge of the disk. This roughness on the cranial surface of the disk is encountered particularly frequently at advanced ages (Müller 1990: 147).

Another factor, which Müller considers significant, could be adhesions that have developed in the upper region of the disk. I assume that at least some of the morphological changes within the mandibular joint described by Müller are caused by the long-term effects of pressure and tension forces. The forces acting here are caused by structures that intersect the exterior of the joint or by structures that are involved on an intracapsular level in the normal displacement of the articular disk that occurs during movement of the jaw when the mouth is opened and closed.

Biomechanics of the mandibular joint

The mandibular joint is a "suspended" hinge joint, a functional "hybrid," so to speak; it is held in a type of "base position" by the basic tone of active muscles in conjunction with fascial tension and tendon and ligamentous structures. On the muscular level, this position is primarily guaranteed by three muscles, the temporalis, masseter, and medial pterygoid muscles.

For each function, the mandible moves through a characteristic spatial curve. During the first phase of opening the mouth, a purely joint axis movement normally occurs around the approximately horizontal axis of the joint. During this movement— we are talking about opening the mouth only a few millimeters—the head of the mandible tilts in the anterior direction. In order to allow this tilting movement, the three "holding muscles" of the mandible listed above must passively lengthen. The tension pattern of the temporalis muscle plays an important role here because its fibers are able to induce various directions of movement: the fibers

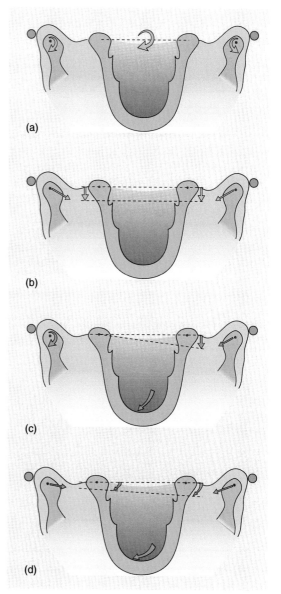

(a)

(b)

(c)

(d)

Figure 7.2 Normal movement pattern of the mandibular joint. (a) Beginning of opening the mouth up to a maximum of 12 mm; rotational movement around the hinge axis of the joint. (b) Continuation of opening the mouth by bilateral protrusion. (c) Unilateral protrusion: the head of the mandibular joint remains mostly in the initial position on one side while a protrusion movement is occurring on the other side. This causes a lateral deviation of the mandible in relation to the vertical center line while the mouth is opened. (d) After the initial hinge axis movement, protrusion now occurs on both sides, with one side moving farther forward than the other.

in the posterior–inferior part of the muscle run almost horizontally, in the center part they run diagonally, and in the frontal portion almost vertically. The temporal muscle has a very peculiar origin that is subdivided in three dimensions. With its deep layers, it originates from the temporal line inferior of the temporal plane, i.e. a "normal" origin on the periosteum of the bone. At the same time, however, its superficial layer originates on the exterior sheath layer, the temporal fascia and its connection with the galea aponeurotica. In addition, the muscle has other attachments in its course in the anterior direction: on the temporal face of the sphenoid bone and on the posterior side of the zygomatic bone. Finally, there is still the variant of an additional tissue fixation when the fascial sheath of the temporal muscle is conjoined with the fascial sheath of the masseter muscle.

Thanks to its three-dimensional origin, the temporalis muscle is able to perform two functions:

- hold the mandible against the maxilla and move the mandible toward the maxilla
- allow grinding motion during mastication.

In order to understand this movement in its spatial process, it is helpful to examine the normal movement pattern in its process over time.

Treatment of the mandibular joint

It is typical of normal joint function for the mandible to be able to perform each of these four movement steps without pain or side noise. A six-step technique will be described below that is suitable for general improvement of joint function and, in particular, for correction of the lack of protrusion. This technique is not appropriate for the treatment of severe, degenerative changes or inflammatory processes. The mandibular joint is very susceptible to tension from all segments of the body. For this reason, it is necessary to prepare for the technique described below by treating the significant restrictions of movement in the organism as a whole. Peculiarly, this sort of restriction of movement may be present in quite diverse sections of the myofascial system and the ligaments and sheaths of the organs. Therefore, an examination of the entire organism using general listening (see Chapter 8) is always

advisable before beginning specialized treatment of the mandibular joint. This sort of preliminary treatment can be applied to various sections of the body.

First step   Treatment of the thoracocervical transition

The goal of this technique is to reduce tension patterns in the region of the clavicle, the subclavius muscle, and the first rib.

Patient   In the dorsal position, legs bent, arms lying next to the torso.

Therapist   Sitting at the head.

Contact   With the fingertips of one hand on the lower edge of the clavicle; with the surface of the second phalanx of the other hand in the lateral region of the neck next to the lateral boundary of the trapezius muscle.

Action   Before the application of this technique, it is necessary to examine the sternoclavicular joint in motion on both sides. On the side where we find a restriction of movement in the upper chest cavity, the therapist's hand surrounds the lower edge of the clavicle in the direction of the subclavius muscle and is elastic against the tissue while pushing the clavicle against the sternum (the patient's left side in the picture). At the same time, the neck is flexed passively to the side and rotated so that the superficial layers (platysma and sternocleidomastoid muscles) relax. It should now be possible to effortlessly make contact in the direction of the middle scalene muscle (the patient's right side in the picture). In the figure, it is visible how the therapist uses the surface of the second phalanx to produce an intensive contact with the middle layer of the neck by reaching inward at the anterior edge of the trapezius muscle. It is crucial that the therapist's left and right hands be moving slightly diagonally relative to one another. The patient's breathing motion will give us information about the activity of the scalene muscles. This technique should be performed as a comparison between sides, for which purpose we use the hands on opposite sides.

With some skill, this technique allows us to treat the structures of the fascial network that run longitudinally and diagonally through the neck. The technique described above can be applied in

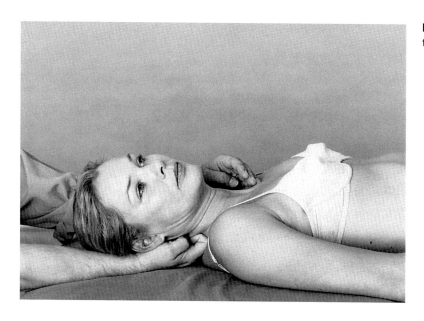

Figure 7.3   Treatment of the thoracocervical transition.

a modified fashion for treating the layer that branches off from the scalene fascia and ends on the upper portion of the pleural cupula (application after whiplash in an automobile accident with a seatbelt).

Second step   Simultaneous influence on the exterior and interior structure of the cranium in the region of the sagittal suture

Patient   In the dorsal position, legs bent, arms lying next to the torso.

Therapist   Sitting at the head.

Contact   With both thumbs in the galea aponeurotica on both sides of the sagittal suture.

Action   Before applying this technique, we first examine the general mobility of the cranium. We test whether the seam of the bone can be elastically compressed by feeling along the entire suture beginning at the anterior edge. While doing so, we should bear in mind that there are considerable variations in the course of the seams of the skull. In the posterior region, the peaks of the seam are broader and allow a greater "spring effect." In this test, the point of the strongest restriction of movement is localized and the exterior fascial and interior membrane fixation located behind it is evaluated on this basis.

As soon as we have localized the point described above, we can now act simultaneously on the exterior sheath structure and the interior membrane structure: we produce an intensive contact with the galea aponeurotica and compress the skull seam, which is already quite "interlocked" at this point, while we maintain intensive contact with the exterior sheath layer as if to loosen the galea aponeurotica from the layer located below it. We wait briefly until a strong counterpressure becomes discernible. As a rule, this occurs within a few seconds. We observe and follow the reactions in the lateral portion of the cranium until our thumbs are pressed upward and apart.

It is important to take into account the asymmetries in the head, both when compressing and also when slowly releasing and also to follow the opening slowly outward so as to be able to affect the interior and exterior layers at the same time.

If, in spite of strong tension in the cranium, no counterpressure occurs, we slightly raise the head and modify the direction of pressure toward the foramen magnum, while continuing to hold the suture compressed. In so doing, we align the pressure as if to push into the vertebral canal through the interior of the head using the foramen magnum, until increased pressure acts from the inside on the sagittal suture and we can feel our two contact points being literally pushed apart.

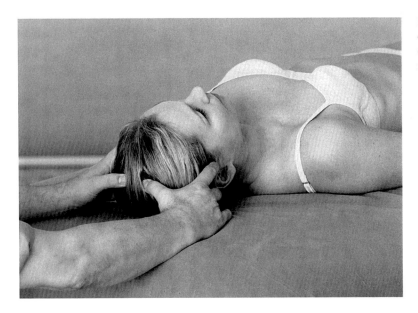

Figure 7.4   Simultaneous influence on the exterior and interior structure of the cranium in the region of the sagittal suture.

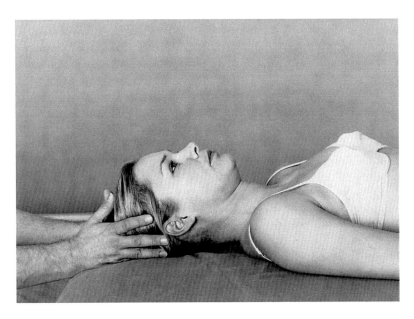

Figure 7.5   Treatment of the fascial layer of the temporalis muscle.

Third step   Treatment of the fascial layer of the temporalis muscle

Patient   In the dorsal position, legs bent, arms lying next to the torso.

Therapist   Sitting at the head.

Contact   With the surface of the fingers of both hands bilaterally in the posterior region of the temporalis muscle.

Action   At first, we feel along the entire origin of the temporalis muscle until we find layers that are particularly closely connected to the bones located below them or to the galea aponeurotica running above them. It is at these points—they may be located at a different place on either side—that we make gentle contact.

We ask the patient to slowly open the mouth and then close it; this allows us to ascertain whether

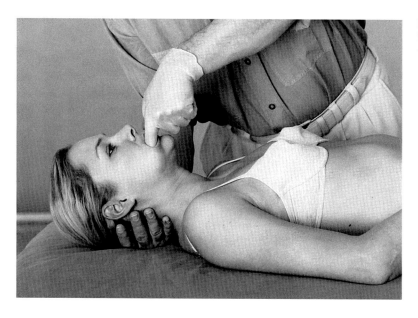

Figure 7.6 Treatment of the insertion of the temporal muscle on the mandible.

parts of the muscle are permanently contracted and whether the fascia has thickened. It is frequently possible to discover a layer on one side that feels considerably denser than the comparable layer on the other side.

We exert a subtle pull in the cranial direction (parallel to the treatment table). Although we are maintaining intensive contact with the temporalis fascia, we should not pull on the bone; rather, we should act on the layers surrounding it in such a way that the bone can find its appropriate mobility. The goal of this technique is to improve the opening function of both mandibular joints.

Fourth step   Treatment of the insertion of the temporalis muscle on the mandible

Patient   In the dorsal position, legs extended, arms lying next to the torso.

Therapist   Standing to the side at the level of the patient's pectoral girdle.

Contact   One hand is supporting the occiput; the tip of the index finger of the other hand contacts the insertion of the temporalis muscle intraorally.

Action   If a permanent contraction of one side of the mandibular joint has occurred, the tensile forces will manifest at the point at which the connective

tissue sheaths of the temporalis muscle meet the periosteum of the mandible. If the tensile forces are permanently present, the insertion point of the temporal muscle on the mandible will feel distinctly hardened. In this case, it is always worthwhile to produce a "melting" touch contact at the connection point between the muscular fascia and periosteum until the fingers producing the contact receive the impression that the bone has received sufficient freedom of movement within the tissue.

Fifth step   Treatment of the spatial relationship between the maxilla, the base of the skull, and the neck

Patient   In the dorsal position, legs bent, arms lying next to the torso.

Therapist   Sitting at the head.

Contact   With one palm in the region of the occiput on the nuchal ligament; with the index and middle fingers of the other hand intraorally in the center section of the palate.

Action   The goal of this treatment is to guarantee that both halves of the maxilla provide adequate orientation as the stable pole of the mandibular joint while the internal membrane lining and exterior fascial layer of the base of the skull display equivalent tension patterns.

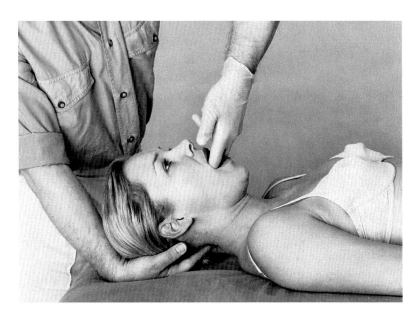

Figure 7.7 Treatment of the spatial relationship between the maxilla, the base of the skull, and the neck.

The precondition for such a global and, at the same time, detailed strategy is that the therapist use one hand to produce intensive contact with the origin of the nuchal ligament on the occiput without compressing the intracranial cavity in the process. The ligament originates as a large surface from the occiput and is attached to each of the posterior processes of the cervical spine before it ends in the fascia of the trapezius muscle. It is essential that we not limit the dynamics of the base of the skull. In other words, all tension modifications that become evident at the occiput during our treatment will be followed but not inhibited. As soon as the supporting hand has found sufficient contact with the occiput, we adapt the index and middle fingers of the other hand intraorally to the form of the center of the palate and create a spatially tangible connection between the two hands. While the occiput remains stable, it is important to sense the dynamics of both halves of the maxilla: it is as if we were placing our hands below two wings of an airplane and pushing against them in order to gradually stretch inflexible membrane layers (the wings) until the impression arises of an even spatial distribution of forces.

During this process, we should bear in mind that "normal" mobility of the bones in tissue is not forced: the index and middle fingers of the intra-oral hand come into intensive and, at the same time, slightly elastic contact with the center section of the palate. As soon as one half of the palate moves, the contact finger follows it. If a twisting of the two halves occurs axially, we can "exaggerate" it without risk until the "wings" of the maxilla find a harmonic movement.

Sixth step   Correction of reduced or absent protrusion on one side

This treatment step has proven itself in practice in cases in which the push is reduced on one side. In such cases, drastic deviation occurs from the center line when the mouth is spontaneously opened.

Patient   In the dorsal position, legs extended, arms lying next to the torso.

Therapist   Standing to the side at the level of the patient's pectoral girdle.

Contact   With the thumb and middle finger on the frontal bone; the little finger of the other hand intraorally parallel to the course of the lateral pterygoid muscle.

Action   In order to reduce the tissue tension that is responsible for the lateral deviation, we must attempt to position the little finger used for treatment as high as possible next to the lateral pterygoid muscle. While the therapist's little finger glides

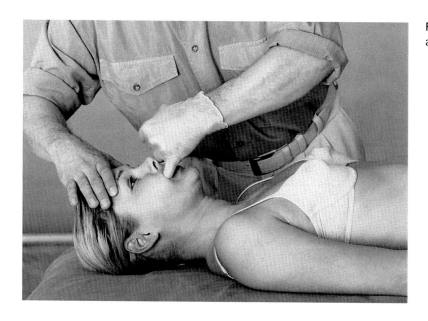

Figure 7.8 Correction of reduced or absent protrusion on one side.

gradually higher and higher, we ask the patient again to open the mouth a few millimeters and then to close it (without the teeth touching each other). The little finger used for treatment finally attains the highest possible position. At this moment, we ask the patient to energetically close the bite while the finger providing the treatment exerts a stretching force on the deep tissue structures around the joint like a wedge.

This treatment directly affects the pterygotemporomandibular aponeurosis. It is helpful to envision the spatial relationship between the lingual and alveolar nerves between the medial pterygoid and lateral pterygoid muscles so as not to press the nerve against the jawbone. Subsequently, we should repeat treatment step 5 again and examine the cervicocranial transition.

TREATMENT AFTER IMPLANTATION OF IMPLANTS IN THE REGION OF THE MAXILLA

In the last 20 years, oral implantology has become considerably more widespread. If the procedures are conducted in an appropriate and careful manner, long-term negative reactions in the craniosacral system are extremely rare. However, one exception is the so-called minimally invasive sinus lift

technique according to Summers, in which a regional lift of the base of the maxillary sinus is performed with circumscribed small fractures of the lamellated bone of the base of the maxillary sinus with the aid of condensation instruments (round bit 1–5 mm in diameter). Here, even if the procedure is conducted correctly and carefully, irritations of the craniosacral system can occur. Depending on the therapist, irritating sensations may occur in 1 to 3 percent of cases.[5]

The low percentage of complications should in no way be taken for granted. I would like to make reference to reports during the meeting of the Bavarian Society of Implantology (Bayerischer Landesverband Implantologie) on April 19–20, 2002, in Würzburg. In contributions to the discussion, it became clear that some implantologists assume a significantly higher percentage of complications.

Schmidinger assumes that the number of problematic implants is very low if the implantologist has the appropriate surgical experience, but

---

[5] I have obtained these numbers from Sebastian Schmidinger, who has performed this technique on over 600 patients. I would like to thank him for his willingness to discuss critically the few complications in his own practice. Over the years, he has given me the opportunity to use manual diagnostics to examine complicated cases and test treatment options.

irritations that may occur in the cranial region should be taken seriously in any event. Moreover, he assumes that implantology, even though it is a minimally invasive procedure, sometimes can cause lasting changes in the area of membrane tension and osseous suture connections in the region of the cranium.

Anatomy of the palatine bone

The primary function of the maxilla is to form a partition between the maxillary and nasal sinuses in order to allow pressure differentials and thus guarantee swallowing and breathing processes independently of one another. This function of the maxilla is essential to life and is already present at birth. The teeth and their alveolar processes do not appear until later.

In the posterior region of the palate, this bone is only a few tenths of a millimeter thick.

In the figure, it is visible that the maxilla is a divided bone that consists of four primary bones. The visible seam of the palate remains even in old age. From the preparation shown, we can see that the alveolar processes are disposed in such a

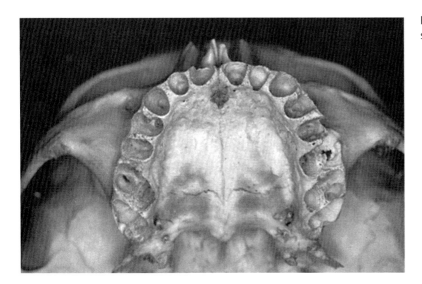

Figure 7.9 Interior view of the bone structure of the palate.

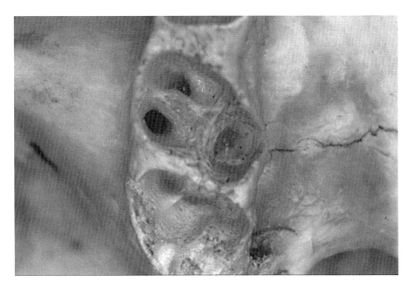

Figure 7.10 Alveolar process of the sixth tooth in the region of the right maxilla.

way that they are at a particular angle to the actual roof of the palate on the palatine surface. This angle causes a stiffening in the region of the alveolar processes and thus a functionally correct adaptation of the bone to the conditions of the bite function. From the fine structures in which the tooth is embedded, we can see how force effects influence the direction of the trabeculae and bone structures.

The alveola consists of relatively little material, but can endure enormous pressure thanks to its fundamental structural principle: experimentally, forces up to 2000 newtons have been measured when biting on a molar tooth. The alveolar process can disintegrate under the influence of inflammatory and atrophic processes.

However, the disintegration of the alveolar processes leaves the center of the maxilla untouched.

The inner edge of the palate is completely preserved; in other words, there is no palatine change. The disintegration is merely limited to regions in which teeth have been lost. This process is particularly visible in the picture in the region of the left canine and the fourth tooth. We can see here that, even in the advanced stages of tooth loss, the uppermost structural principle of the maxilla is

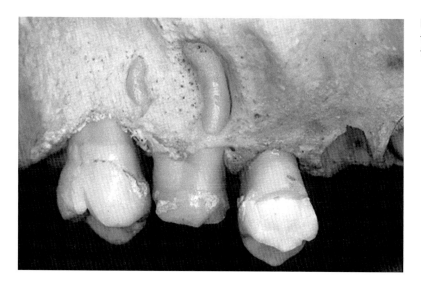

Figure 7.11   Disintegration process in the region of the alveolar processes of the maxilla.

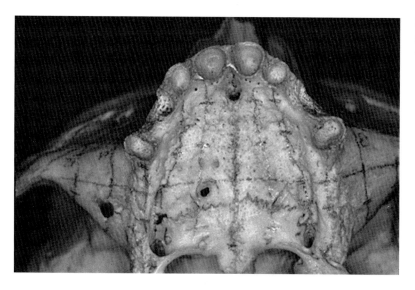

Figure 7.12   Preparation with advanced disintegration in the region of the alveolar processes.

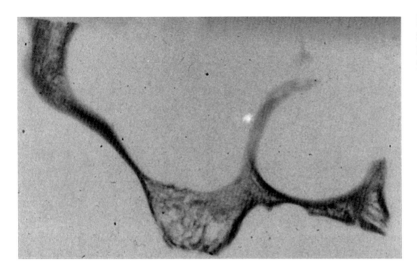

Figure 7.13   Maxillary and nasal sinuses with separating wall. Radiographic cross-section with a thickness of 5 mm of the preparation.

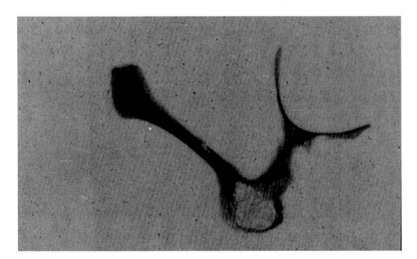

Figure 7.14   Changed bone structure in the preparation of a diabetic.

maintained, namely to form a partition between two cavities.

The bones that separate the two cavities from one another are a razor-thin structure.

Under the influence of diabetes, the trabeculae are rarefied; very little cancellous bone still remains. The individual laminar layers are thickened.

Technique of the surgical intervention

In a sinus lift, the implantologist opens the maxillary sinus from the ventral or lateral side. In so doing, the mucous membrane, known as Schneider's membrane, is guided in the cranial direction using a round bit.

Lifting Schneider's membrane is technically necessary in order to create a space between the membrane and the osseous base of the maxillary sinus so that the implant can be inserted.

When opening the maxillary sinus, the implantologist is forced to work with a round bit, tapping in the cranial direction. This can lead to changes in the region of the sutures of the maxilla and adjacent bones. However, it is also conceivable that transmissions of vibrations could cause a dysfunction of the membranous equilibrium of the craniosacral system located at a distance from the

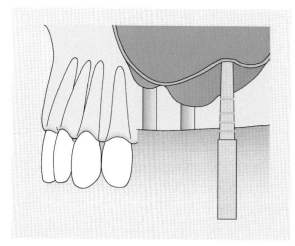

Figure 7.15 Opening the maxillary sinus and lifting Schneider's membrane in the cranial direction.

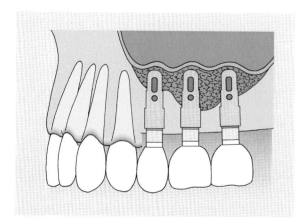

Figure 7.16 Placing three implants in the region of the maxilla.

point of the surgical intervention. Schmidinger assumes that, in some cases, the implantologist may be reinforcing or possibly even creating displacements of the spatial axes of movement of the craniosacral system.[6]

---

[6] Contribution by Sebastian Schmidinger to discussion after my talk on the effects of sinus and elevation techniques on the craniosacral system at the meeting of the Bavarian Society of Implantology (Bayerischer Landesverband Implantologie) on April 20, 2002, in Würzburg.

Consequences for treatment

It can be clearly seen from the preparations shown that a fine structure is present in the maxilla. In comparison, the mandible is much more massively developed in its osseous structure. It has a thick compacta. In a comparison between the maxilla and mandible, we can see an enormous functional adaptability of tensegrity structures. The maxilla is constructed of fine shells, a lightweight construction, so to speak. These thin osseous lamellae are attached to one another in curved planes. I have already mentioned that, in an individual case, pressure up to 2000 newtons can come into effect when biting. Owing to its lightweight construction, the maxilla is very stiff and therefore able to accept this pressure with minimal elasticity. In contrast, the mandible is deflected when biting down even though it has substantially more massive osseous substance. In a comparison between the maxilla and mandible, the advantages of the "lightweight construction," i.e. the structure having less osseous substance and a plurality of taut membranous components, become clear. However, it also becomes comprehensible why the most minimally invasive intervention by the implantologist can lead in some cases to irritations that must be taken very seriously. I assume that the cause of these irritations is twofold. The first may lie in the fact that, in the case in question, a strong inner twisting of the bone and membrane system is already present in the craniomandibular region. It is possible that an unfavorable rhythm in tapping with the condensation instrument is sufficient to establish the existing twisted distortion for good, so to speak. As a second possible cause, we must consider that too massive an application of the round bit completely traumatizes the cranial system. However, it could also be that all too gentle tapping by the overly careful implantologist could imperceptibly sneak its way into the fluctuations of pressure in the craniosacral fluid system, so to speak, and unintentionally throw the entire tension system of the intracranial membranes into disarray.

For manual treatment, it is necessary to examine the mobility of all of the sutures; in other words, not only in the region of the maxilla. The general tension behavior of the dura should also be tested in the entire area between the cranium and sternum. In any event, I recommend first treating the

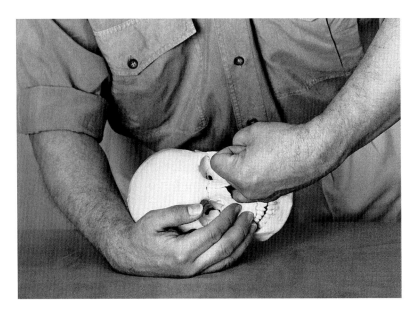

Figure 7.17   Hand position in the region of the right maxilla and nasal cavity.

restrictions of movement that manifest in the neurocranium and only then continue with the treatment of the viscerocranium.[7]

If a restriction of motion is found in the maxilla or especially on one side of the maxilla, initially treating the spatial relationships between the maxilla, base of the skull, and neck as I described in the preceding section (Fascial technique for the treatment of the mandibular joint) is advisable.

Sometimes it is possible to diagnose an almost absolute restriction of motion of the maxilla on the side where the implant was placed in the maxilla. In such a case, the affected half appears to be completely rigid as soon as we exert pressure on it while the other side gives way under pressure in a very elastic fashion. As a rule, this is caused by a global fixation of the membranes on one side of the cranium with a simultaneous "pressure interlock" in one half of the maxilla.

Treatment of unilateral restriction of motion of the maxilla

Patient   Prone, with the head rotated to the side such that the part of the maxilla to be treated is resting on the treatment table.

---

[7]See the description of treatment of the sutures of the skull in Liem (1998: 510–35).

Therapist   Standing to the side at the head.

Contact   When treating the right half of the maxilla, the therapist supports the maxilla on this side from outside, while at the same time placing the little finger of the other hand into the nasal cavity using a water-soluble lubricant gel.

Action   The weight of the patient's head is allowed to rest on the therapist's right hand. The contact point is approximately in the region of the roots of the left premolars of the maxilla.

The little finger of the left hand, the treatment finger, is in a vinyl glove that is coated with lubricant gel. This finger is very gently inserted into the nasal cavity parallel to the nasal septum. Here, it is important that it be guided not in the superior direction toward the eye, but rather parallel to the arch of the palate. The therapist thus uses the little finger to make contact with the bone and membrane structure of the mandibular cavity by way of the nasal cavity while supporting the lateral osseous boundary of the same region from the outside. The therapist uses the weight of the cranium so as to guide the entire fine bone structure of the maxilla more intensely into its twisted distortion. At the endpoint of this movement, the therapist applies a slow pull—albeit with lasting effect—in the interior of the nasal cavity until the movement of the maxilla begins to emerge.

In this procedure, it is important to precisely detect the very fine bone structure between the nasal cavity and mandibular cavity and use the membrane tensions connected to it to examine the resilient elasticity. A painful procedure in the region of the nasal cavity should be avoided under all circumstances. This technique is also suitable for the treatment of mechanical traumas in the region of the viscerocranium.

After the unilateral mobilization technique on the maxilla, I recommend repeating the treatment of the spatial relationship between the maxilla, base of the skull, and neck (step 5). The unilateral correction technique described here is also "minimally invasive" to a certain extent. For the purpose of achieving a stable treatment result, a final treatment of the atlanto-occipital connection (see section 5.1, Treatment of the atlanto-occipital connection) and the transition between the sacrum and lumbar spine (see section 5.1, Decompression technique for the transition between the lower lumbar spine and sacrum) is also advisable.

Chapter 8

Treatment of the fascial and membrane system after whiplash

Mechanics of whiplash

In whiplash, acceleration forces act in an abrupt manner on the human body and may have impact on the entire connective tissue system. Here, the extent of the forces at work is not necessarily an indicator of the damage caused. We know from practice that there are high-speed traumas with multiple fractures that leave the basic structure of the fascial and membrane system relatively undamaged, while it is sometimes the effect of relatively small forces, if they are acting from a certain unfavorable angle, that can create lasting problems from which the organism is no longer able to free itself.

It is a complication for diagnostics that most of the changes that occur to connective tissue due to whiplash cannot be seen using imaging procedures. As a result, it is all too easy to push into the psychological field symptoms that are unbearable for patients. I do not believe that the psychological side of certain types of trauma should be disregarded—even in traffic accidents where no injuries occur, there is the potential for psychoemotional complications. As a rule, however, accidents of this sort are a primarily mechanical event that extends into the interior, interconnected structure of the entire organism. The physical changes can be complicated by the psychological reaction, but they still require treatment on a physical level if they can be clearly diagnosed.

As mentioned at the outset, forces in whiplash act on the body in a very abrupt fashion. This can be caused by acceleration, but also by deceleration or stopping. In order to understand the effect of this process, it is helpful to consider again the properties of membranes and fasciae.

We have described it as a characteristic of this type of tissue (Chapter 2, The malleability of connective tissue) that it has a certain degree of elasticity and plasticity. These characteristics are typical of all forms of connective tissue. In whiplash, demands are placed on both characteristics of the connective tissue: the sudden effect of acceleration forces causes the layers that have primarily elastic components to be stretched in a particularly lasting manner, while the very tough layers are able to resist this stretching to a large extent. Because collagen fibers have a maximum extensibility of 5 to 10 percent, they guarantee that the basic shape of the organism is maintained even under the influence of strong forces (e.g. in the case of high-speed trauma). Nevertheless, the effects of a minor, lasting deformation of these tough fibrous layers should not be underestimated. However, the more lasting deformation occurs in the layers that contain a high percentage of elastin. This is true not only for layers of connective tissue in the literal sense, but also for individual ligaments such as the ligamentum flavum and nuchal ligament.

In order for the connective tissue to be able to perform its function, the shape-maintaining collagen fibers must cooperate with the elastic elements. Changes in form may be reversed using the elastic fibers. The elastin returns to its own "resting length" and, in so doing, guides the less elastic elements back to their original position before the stretching process. However, during an accident, the elastin is stretched beyond its limit of elasticity. This means that the spatially changed, low-elasticity fibers are also unable to reach their original position. A lasting displacement and deformation of the inner form structure of the organism ensues.

In the literature, the deformability of elastic layers is described as irreversible as long as the original length of a tissue unit has been increased over one and a half times (150 percent). In whiplashes, this increase in length can be exceeded many times over. In high-speed traumas, individual layers are overstretched even up to ten times their original extension. This can result in a lasting alteration process of the entire inner fundamental blueprint of the organism, which can influence not only movement functions, but also a number of other bodily functions such as the metabolic and endocrine processes, for example.

Examination of whiplash

In every case, an orthopedic examination should be made first in order to rule out any fractures that would prohibit manual treatment for the time being. Sometimes a neurological examination is advisable as well. In the case of the most severe traumas, possible ligamentous ruptures between the upper cervical vertebrae and the base of the skull should be considered as well. As soon as the traditional medical examinations have been concluded, a general manual examination may be performed. When doing so, it is important to bear in mind that, in cases of whiplash, we are confronted not only with current results of the accident, but also with problems that existed beforehand. The state of the organism before the accident is usually reinforced and made worse by the mechanical influences. Whiplash has a particularly lasting effect at the points where restrictions of movement or degenerative changes were already present. In a way, this also explains why a relatively small force can cause lasting problems in one case whereas, in a different case, the same degree of force leaves no effect on the organism. The significance of the state of the organism before the accident, known as the "prelesional state," as Barral and Croibier have called it, cannot be emphasized enough (Barral and Croibier 1999: 184–90).

Fundamentally, deformations of the fascial and membrane system are possible in all regions of this three-dimensional network. Details can be changed, or a global deformation process can be set into motion, which is initially quite diffused and is difficult diagnostically to categorize to individual layers or joints. Unfortunately, the conversion processes associated with global deformation have a negative and progressive dynamic that can extend over long periods of time, months and sometimes years. I have already mentioned that the state of the patient is crucial for the positive treatment capacity of our treatment principles. In general, we should direct our attention to peculiarities of this preceding situation. In particular, arthrotic changes in the cervical spine, intervertebral disk problems in all regions of the spine, and healed fractures all require us to proceed very carefully. This is also true of neurological problems that existed before the accident and may have been made worse by the effect of whiplash forces.

It is helpful to precisely study the circumstances of the accident, if available, in order to understand the peculiarities of the effects of the forces to which the organism was subjected. For example, a driver whose stationary automobile was hit from behind by another vehicle will suffer from a different whiplash than a passenger in a vehicle in a frontal collision. Different forces are experienced by the body of an airline passenger in a descending airplane during turbulence than by a mountain climber who freefalls several meters to be caught by a safety rope. Knowledge of the exterior conditions is important because there are very specific constellations that can be classified as presenting particular problems from the outset. The direction from which the force acts on the person's body plays an important role. In my practice, I have found an especially large number of complications in cases in which the primary shear force acted on the organism from the side, such as in automobile accidents in which one vehicle is hit from the side by the active impact force of another vehicle. It is of importance whether the occupants of a vehicle saw the other vehicle in the accident coming toward them. The driver will then reflexively step on the brake and, in a fraction of a second, the first force will act on the lower extremity, whose musculature is strongly contracted. This causes a massive jerking shear force to act on the pelvis. This shear force damages the ligaments of joints and the organs of the pelvis. However, longitudinal displacements of the two bones of the lower leg relative to one another or articular fixations in the region of the ankle and metatarsus frequently occur as well.

If the patient is in pain, the manual examination must be conducted in such a way as to avoid intensifying the pain. In any event, one should avoid direct stretching in the examination. The position of the patient's body should be selected so that it is resting in as pain-free a position as

possible and any vertigo the patient may experience should not be intensified by the selected position or changes to it. It is sometimes necessary to examine the patient only in a sitting or standing position. If the patient is lying down, care should be taken that the cervical spine is not overextended. Because multiple injuries always occur in a complex whiplash, it is crucial that the therapist precisely localize the few central changes and correctly evaluate their significance. Only in this way will we be able to prevent stress that sometimes causes further irritation by treating the compensatory side aspects. In certain cases of whiplash, the entire body is in a constant state of irritation. A less specific treatment process that desires to reach many different elements of the organism can cause more damage than it heals. This can cause an unconscious resistance to further treatment on the part of the patient, which can disrupt the healing process.

Problem zones

As a result of the immense shear and tensile forces that act on the human organism in cases of whiplash, lasting changes in tension can occur in all components of the organism. In order to recognize the primary restrictions from the outset, it is helpful during examination to direct our attention to the problem zones which are affected frequently and in a particularly lasting manner:

- ligamentous injuries in the region of the ankle and metatarsus and associated restrictions of movement in the joints
- longitudinal displacement of the tibia and fibula
- changes to the ligaments between the sacrum and ilium, especially with consequences for the lower part of the joint connection of the iliosacral joint
- restriction of the sacrococcygeal joint
- restrictions of motion of organs and global changes to the connective tissue beds
- restrictions of motion in joints of the spine
- restrictions within the sternum and adjacent structures, in particular retrosternal structures

- restrictions of the sternoclavicular joint in connection with changes of tone in the subclavicular layers
- changes to the tensile force between the dura mater and the components of the body connected to it
- changes to the various tissue layers of the suboccipital triangle
- changes to the mobility of the cranial sutures, particularly in the base of the skull
- changes to the membranous connection between the maxilla and the skull bones located above it
- changes in the region of the mandibular joint.

This is not a complete list; it only names the aspects that, as a rule, are at the center of the problem. In light of the variety of possible deformations and restrictions of motion, it is recommended to keep the examination very general at the beginning so as to be able to localize the changes of form and motion restrictions that have the greatest significance in whiplash. The general listening and local listening processes originally developed by Pierre Barral are particularly suitable in this case. Both techniques have been accepted for the most part as an important component of osteopathic culture and are also applied outside the osteopathic field. The advantage of this type of examination lies in the fact that the body is touched so carefully that the risk of additional irritation has been eliminated to a large extent. Any oversensitivity of the patient that may manifest is respected and shock-induced reactions can be avoided without a problem. If the therapist is acquainted with Barral's thermal diagnosis, this process should be used to examine the test findings. Because this diagnostic procedure does not use any manual contact, it is particularly suitable for situations in which acute injuries are present. The temperature differentials that can be detected in thermal diagnosis can usually be perceived without a problem. Precise categorization regarding individual anatomical structures requires extraordinary sensitivity and the most precise, detailed anatomical knowledge (Barral 1996).

General listening in the standing position (according to Barral)

Patient   Standing with the legs slightly apart.

Therapist   Standing behind the patient.

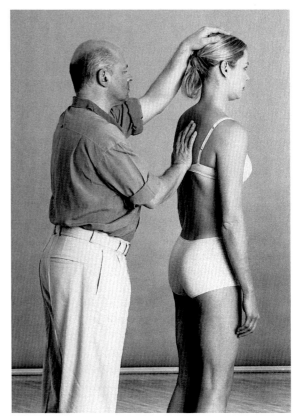

Figure 8.1   General listening in the standing position.

Contact   With the flat hand on the cap of the skull.

Action   The therapist places one hand on the cap of the skull and asks the patient to close his or her eyes; the therapist's hand is completely relaxed and does not exert any active pressure. The therapist's attention is now directed at whether the tensile force acting under this hand is emitting in a particular direction. Here, it is important for the therapist's attention to be entirely centered on the interior of the palm and not on the tactile contact of the fingers. If this technique is applied correctly, the patient will be able to tell whether a connection has been created between the therapist's testing hand and the primary problem zone.

General listening in the sitting position (according to Barral)

Patient   Sitting.

Therapist   Standing behind the patient.

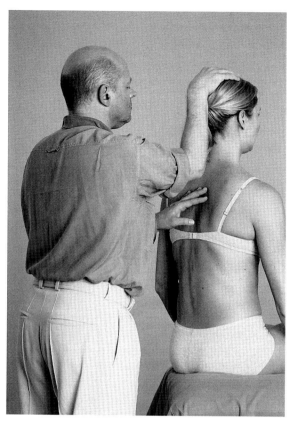

Figure 8.2   General listening in the sitting position.

Contact   With the palm of the hand on the cap of the skull.

Action   The therapist's hand is used in the same manner as in the technique described above. Because the region of the lower extremities is excluded from the observational field of the test by the sitting position, the test result found in the standing position may be made more precise. It is advisable to supplement this test with the following test for the region of the chest cavity and the shoulders.

General listening in the sitting position from the anterior side (according to Barral)

Patient   Sitting.

Therapist   Sitting in front of the patient.

Contact   With both forearms under the patient's slightly raised forearms.

Action   The therapist makes sure to have good contact with the floor and to be sitting neither in a slouched position nor overly erect. Using the palms of the hands and the forearm, the therapist accepts the weight of the patient's arms and now pays attention to whether and in which direction a pull impulse can be felt on one side. This pull impulse is a sign of the side on which we will find the restriction.

> In performing the general listening technique, there is the risk that the therapist will project processes from his or her own organism onto the patient's body by way of the tactile senses. This can be best prevented by the therapist being in an equilibrium of the autonomic nervous system. In other words, the therapist should not be in an overactive state or in a greatly relaxed state. The watchword for "listening" is "quiet attention."

Skeptics may note that examinations of this type are actually very vague and should not be taken seriously by science in comparison with the "objectivity" of the examination of joints in the musculoskeletal system. We can respond to these skeptics by saying that, when we examine a joint, we touch the bone itself only in the rarest of cases and the bones that are easier to touch are part of a model that, while it arises from a certain reasonable, schematized viewpoint, is in no way more "real" than the tensile forces that are tangible in the myofascial system. In order to understand the meaning and capacity of the "listening" process, we must merely compare it with other sensory perceptions. The musician's skilled ear registers the sound of each individual instrument of the orchestra and, with the inner ear, can even hear the true tone of transposed instruments from a score, which would be difficult or even incomprehensible for musical laypersons. I think that general listening is a sort of tactile hearing. The therapist's hand registers and localizes the course of the movement curves in the interior of the patient's organism in the same manner in which the musician registers the course of the rhythm and melody of individual instruments.

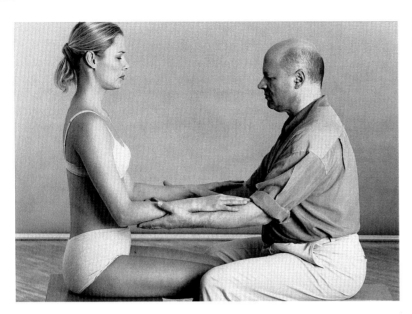

Figure 8.3　General listening in the sitting position from the anterior side.

Alternative test to Barral's general listening

Patient　In the dorsal position, legs extended with the ankles reaching just over the edge of the treatment table.

Therapist　Sitting at the foot.

Contact　With both hands from the posterior direction in the lower third of the calves.

Action　Both of the therapist's feet are in good contact with the floor and the therapist's posture is neither slouched nor overly erect. The object is for the therapist's posture to be contributed by the organ column and the autonomic musculature while the exterior musculature of the ribcage and pectoral girdle are relaxed. The weight of the therapist's forearms is rested on the treatment table and the therapist's hands hold both calves. The primary weight of the legs is resting on the therapist's palms while the therapist's fingers are relaxed and slightly bent. The therapist now closes his or her eyes in order to aid visualization. The therapist imagines that the two calves are scales resting in his or her hands. The therapist then adjusts the touch of these scales so that it has precisely the same quality on both sides. This means that the therapist's hand has been adapted on each side to the existing shape of the right or left calf. Now the therapist gradually exerts a subtle but very steady shear force along the inner longitudinal axis of the legs in the direction of

the pelvis. The therapist first feels whether a resistance to the shear force manifests inside the leg, for example at the level of the knee or at the transition to the pelvis. This is a sign of an injury or restriction on the side in question. It is possible to avoid the resistance and continue with the test if the therapist slightly reduces the shear force and then successively intensifies it again as if to slowly turn up the dimmer on a light switch. Thus, the therapist is gradually able to transmit the shear force into the interior of the pelvic and abdominal cavities and the area can be localized in which resistance is occurring. In this area as well, we first reduce the shear force somewhat as soon as we encounter resistance and then gently intensify it again and transmit it through the diaphragm into the interior of the chest cavity. As a rule, as soon as we are pushing against the diaphragm, we must wait for a moment because the force we are applying is initially transmitted by way of the arch of the diaphragm into the prevertebral space of the central tendon.

In the most favorable case, we will be able to continue the shear test into the region of the neck and cranium. This test is primarily suitable for localizing severe restrictions in the region of the ligamentous connections of the organs by sensing resistance to the subtle push. This technique provides little information on restrictions of movement located very close to the middle central axis of the body such as restriction in the joint of the tailbone or

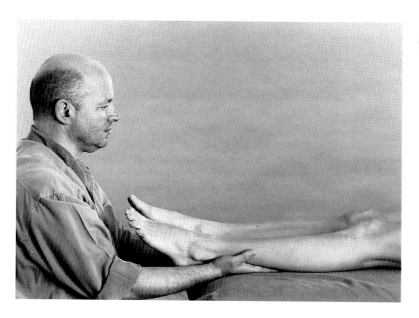

Figure 8.4   Alternative test to Barral's general listening.

sacrum or the large longitudinal components such as the esophagus and trachea.

Variation of general listening in the dorsal position

Patient   In the dorsal position, legs extended.

Therapist   Sitting at the head.

Contact   With the bent front phalanges of the index, middle, and ring fingers of both hands in the tissue just below the base of the skull.

Action   The therapist first moves the fingertips slightly in the vertical direction in order to intensify the contact with the suboccipital tissue. Then the therapist uses all involved fingertips to pull gently longitudinally through the whole body. In so doing, the therapist precisely observes whether this pull is met with stronger resistance on the left side or right side. On this side, the therapist now precisely differentiates which finger is able to feel the resistance most clearly. We speculate that the localization of the resistance with the ring finger, which is applied in the medial plane, is a sign of fixations in the region of the dura; resistance in the region of the middle finger is a sign of fixations in the region of the organ system; and resistance in the region of the index finger is a sign of fixations in the region of the parietal system. This test procedure is naturally a process that is very difficult to understand rationally. I can only refer to its performance and significance in practice (Prat 1999).

This test can deliver misleading results if unilateral tension patterns are present in the suboccipital region of at the base of the skull. In such a case, it is necessary to differentiate precisely between the local restrictions of the atlanto-occipital connection and the forces acting from a greater distance.

Treatment of whiplash

In cases of whiplash, it is advisable to wait a few days or even a few weeks before the first manual treatment. The reason for waiting lies in the fact that a drastic development of symptoms frequently does not occur until days or weeks after an accident. Especially if the patient has a tendency toward psychological reactions, it is advisable to wait for the first high point of the pain symptoms. If the therapist treats the patient immediately after the accident during a relatively pain-free period of time and the symptoms do not develop in their full scope until after this treatment, the patient will be under the impression that these problems were made

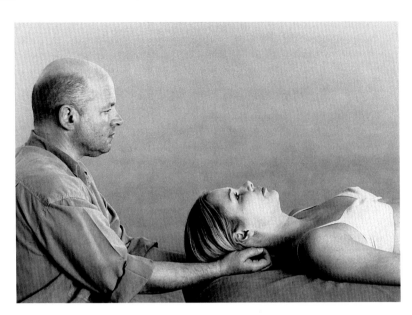

Figure 8.5 General listening in the dorsal position.

worse by the therapy. This will necessarily lead to the development of inner resistance and can considerably complicate the course of treatment. It is also significant that the accident represents a drastic physical development and the possibility that the patient may initially experience any physical treatment on the subconscious level as a continuation of this physical effect cannot entirely be ruled out. For this reason as well, treatment techniques should be selected with the greatest care and it is essential to treat only the problems that can be clearly diagnosed. Too little is better than too much!

In selecting the treatment technique, we should remain strictly within the framework of the injuries and restrictions of movement found in general listening and attempt to reconstruct which portion was already present before the accident and which injuries and restrictions of movement can actually be attributed to the accident. It is helpful to use the most gentle techniques possible, avoiding strong pull effects and abrupt applications of force.

The patient is frequently still in a state of shock even weeks after the accident. This means that the autonomic nervous system is subliminally in a constant state of ergotropic agitation. In addition to the purely physical causes, this is the reason for the sleeplessness that we sometimes observe. For this reason, the therapist must select the quality of the touch in such a way that the manner of treatment normalizes the dynamics between ergotropic and trophotropic activation. In other words, the treatment should first give only minimal stimuli so that, after every agitation of the system, the corresponding relaxation is allowed to emerge. The first touches are crucial.

In practice, we see again and again that, if the lower extremity is carefully treated, a calming of the state of agitation occurs. If changes have occurred in this region, it is advisable to begin treatment there, for example, with a careful correction of restrictions of movement in the region of the ankle or metatarsus. The method that I showed in the section on special joint techniques (see Chapter 6, Special techniques for treating the joints of the foot) is suitable for this purpose.

The usually comprehensive fixation of the dura mater and its tensile effects should be treated in connection with the large anterior longitudinal ligament of the spine. Techniques applied to the sacrum should be used first, and then the treatment should be continued in the region of the cranium.

The essential subsequent step is the treatment of the elements inside the visceral cavities, i.e. the treatment of changes to ligamentous and mesenteric layers of organs.

The mobility of any of the organs may have been affected by the force of the accident. For the first treatment steps in the visceral region, it is crucial to evaluate the transitions between the visceral cavities. Because of the transition between cavities having different hydrostatic pressure, these transitions are particularly at risk because the existing pressure differential may have been increased many times over by the force of the impact. By gliding on their serosal layer and through the overstretching of ligamentous connections, entire organ groups can be spatially displaced. This displacement causes the segments of the body to appear displaced relative to one another on the exterior as well. In such a situation, corrective attempts applied to the parietal system have little effect.

We should give particular attention to the organs located directly below the diaphragm and the retroperitoneal organs or sections of organs, particularly the kidneys. If the victim in an accident was wearing a seat belt, the transition between the chest cavity and the lower cervical region should be precisely examined, particularly in the anterior region. The deep laminae of the neck are frequently affected, as well as the ligamentous suspension of the pleural cupula that connects the central cervical spine to the uppermost section of the endothoracic fascia and thus to the pleural cupula itself.

In whiplash, massive impactions can occur at the sutures of the bones of the skull. However, we should bear in mind that the classic, very subtle craniosacral application in treatment of whiplash has its limits. As much as we should allow our actions in this region to be guided by caution, it is a reality that severe changes may have been caused in the craniosacral region by the accident, requiring a very decisive intervention, otherwise our work in the craniosacral system would produce only a deep relaxation. The relatively drastic techniques of Barral and Croibier, which are primarily directed at the inner elasticity of the bones of the skull, and associated techniques for treating the membranous connections between the maxilla and skull have particularly proven themselves in practice (Barral and Croibier 1999: 184–90, 266–7).

Although these changes that typically occur in whiplash particularly manifest in the area of the neck, extreme restraint is advisable in this section of the body. This is the region where the patient feels the symptoms particularly intensely. If there are restrictions of motion between cervical vertebrae, it is advisable to avoid direct manipulation

for the time being. Direct joint manipulation could have drastic negative consequences from which it takes the patient a long time to recover.

In cases of whiplash, there is frequently a strong emotionalization of which the patient is usually not aware. This emotionalization should be respected for the purpose of a positive course of treatment. On the physical level, it is expressed in tonal chains of the musculature and an individual bodily posture. We should avoid applying so-called myofascial release stretching to the large fascial layers of the system. Rather, the patient should at first have the opportunity to assume the body positions that correspond to the interior expression. Only after the dominant inner fixations have been released will we move the large exterior sheath layers in the direction of the normal pattern.

To give an example, if the organism appears to be slouched, this may be attributable to a restriction of movement in the kidneys. In such a case, an alignment by treating the myofascial layers at the surface would only cause additional discrepancies between the interior structure and the exteriorly visible static of the body. In comparison, a treatment strategy that first makes contact with the entire system by way of the lower extremity and then releases a few restrictions in the interior of the visceral and craniosacral system and only then addresses the autonomic musculature of the back and ribcage is associated with far fewer risks.

Treatment of altered tensile effects of the dura mater by mobilizing the second segment of the sacrum

> If the dura mater is under abnormal tension, the sacrum as a whole appears limited in its movement. The second segment, to which the dura is attached, also appears to be harder than the rest of the bone.

Patient   In the dorsal position, both legs extended.

Therapist   Standing to the side at the level of the thighs.

Contact   Supporting the sacrum from the posterior direction with a flat palm while the other hand supports the lower lumbar spine, also from the posterior direction. The hand position is subsequently switched so as to produce direct contact on the sacrum with the fingertips of both hands.

Action The therapist first takes the sacrum in one hand so as to adapt it to the posterior arch of the bone. At the same time, the other hand is supporting the lower lumbar spine from the posterior direction, but avoids exerting pressure on the spine itself.

At the contact point on the sacrum, the therapist now exerts a pull in the direction of the tailbone without altering the existing tilt of the pelvis or the bend of the lumbar region. In other words, the therapist pulls the sacrum in such a way that the pull acts inward in the vertebral canal and the state of the dura mater can be evaluated. In the case of changes to the tension pattern, the counterpull will manifest at the second segment of the sacrum. The therapist now positions the tips of the fingers and

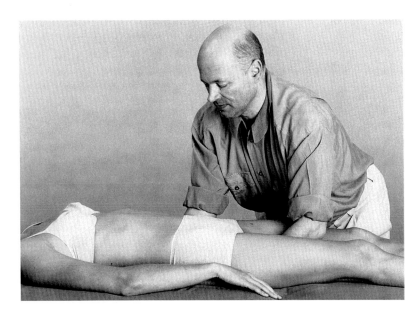

Figure 8.6 Treatment of altered tensile effects of the dura mater by mobilizing the second segment of the sacrum.

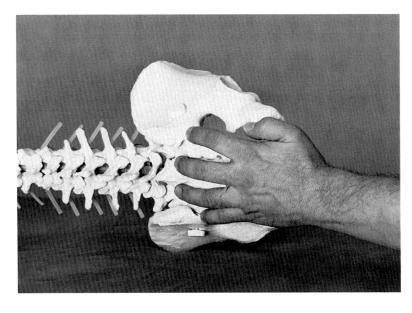

Figure 8.7 Position of the hand on the sacrum.

thumbs around the second segment of the sacrum so that several contact points are produced on the bone. The therapist ensures that the sacrum as a whole is resting on these contact points without changing its position. The therapist now modifies the touch reaching through the subcutaneous layer and lumbar fascia as though to compress the periosteum more strongly against the bone, avoiding any sliding of the surface of the sacrum, and intensifies the contact as if to push through the sheath of the periosteum into the bone. While maintaining this very peculiar type of contact, the therapist feels whether a "melting reaction" is present at the connection points between the tissue and the bone. As a rule, this is a minimal movement that the therapist should follow in all directions until the rigidity at the second segment of the sacrum begins to be released. Subsequently, reassuming the original position of the hands on the sacrum and lumbar region is recommended so as to examine the result of the treatment.

Treatment of the shock pattern in the region of the diaphragm

Patient   In the dorsal position, legs extended.

Therapist   Standing to the side at the level of the thighs.

Contact   With the palms of both hands in and above the region of the twelfth rib from the posterior side, parallel to the course of the ribs.

Action   The therapist registers the breathing movement and compares the right and left sides. On the side where less spatial excursion of the diaphragm can be felt, the therapist successively compresses the posterior chest cavity. During this, it is important that the patient continue to breathe so that several breathing cycles occur during compression. The therapist now begins to use the palm to compress the lower chest cavity on the other side. The therapist maintains the compression of both halves of the thorax and pushes the side that feels freer somewhat more strongly toward the central line while following the direction of the costal arch. This will cause the inner pressure to increase even more on the side of the restriction. The therapist now uses this increase in pressure to release the costal arch and guide it into a greater expansion in the lateral and posterior directions. The therapist's hands are now returned to their initial position in order to compare the spatial excursion of both halves of the diaphragm yet again. If the desired effect is not felt, I recommend waiting a few minutes and then performing the technique again with a slightly different direction of pressure.

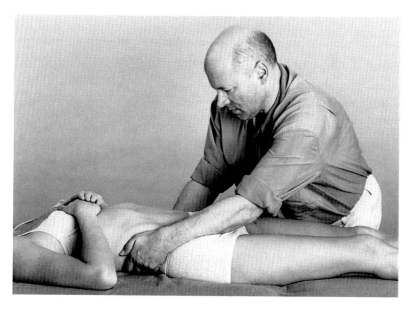

Figure 8.8   Treatment of the shock pattern in the region of the diaphragm.

The variety of layers touching one another at the transition between the chest and abdominal cavities does not always make it easy to definitively determine where exactly our treatment is having its effect. It is certain that this technique affects spasm-like patterns of the diaphragm itself. However, it also affects the connective tissue connection between the organs of the upper abdomen and the diaphragm, and it certainly also has an effect on the distribution of the serosal layer in the narrow gaps between organs. In performing this technique, it is crucial that the therapist compress the intermediate layers of the chest wall from the posterior direction so subtly that it is possible to observe the reaction of the inner components surrounded by these intermediate layers. Based on this observation, the therapist will be able to treat the relatively tough fascial and membrane structure of the ribcage at the same time as the connective tissue sheaths and ligamentous suspensions of the organs they surround. The procedure described by John Upledger (Upledger and Vredevoogd 1983: 46–9) is a suitable alternative or supplement to the treatment described above.

Treatment of the transition between the upper chest cavity and lower cervical region

Patient   In the dorsal position, legs extended.

Therapist   Sitting at the head.

Contact   With the thumbs and fingertips on both sides of the costal joint connections at the level of the fourth thoracic vertebra; the other hand supports the occiput.

Action   The therapist slightly raises the occiput without exerting a pull on the cervical spine. Using the fingers of the other hand, the therapist supports the upper portion of the thoracic region from the posterior direction. At this point, the therapist produces an intensive contact with the relatively superficial fascial layer of the trapezius muscle. In contrast to the muscle fibers, the fibers of the right and left fascia form one unit. The therapist uses the other hand to maintain gentle contact with the origin of the nuchal ligament. If the head and neck want to give way in rotation and lateral flexion, the therapist supports these movements to their endpoint and allows this twisting to remain in the supported position. At the same time, the therapist reaches toward the contact points of the fascial tissue in the upper region of the back, taking care not to glide on the contact points, but rather to apply increased pressure through the deep fascia in the direction of the interior of the body, as if the fingertips were wandering through the patient's body in the direction of the ceiling. As soon as the supporting hand in the region of the back of the head is able to sense that the head wants to return to the central line, the therapist follows this movement. It is crucial that the intensive pressure in the region of the upper chest cavity remain until the movement back to the central line has been completed.

Treatment of the transition between the upper cervical spine and the head

Patient   In the dorsal position, legs extended.

Therapist   Sitting at the head.

Contact   One hand holds the occiput, while the thumb and fingers of the other hand support the space between the second cervical vertebra and the base of the skull on both sides next to the vertebrae.

Action   In this technique, we apply the technique described for the upper chest cavity and lower cervical region (see above) to the very small area of the atlanto-occipital transition. Here as well, it is crucial that the hand placed farther in the inferior direction, i.e. on the neck, be fixed while the hand placed farther in the superior direction on the occiput follow the movement tendencies and thus allow the head to turn or tilt into the position dictated by the dominant tension conditions. The hand supporting the occiput therefore follows in "listening" while the tip of the thumb and fingertips of the other hand hold the myofascial bed of the upper cervical spine. This holding position remains unchanged until a change in tone is discernible and the head moves back to the central line.

The tendency of the head to change its position can still be sensed after the first treatment. The therapist should then support the rotation and lateral flexion movement a second time, and sometimes a third and fourth time. In so doing, the therapist is able to modify the contact in the region of the cervical spine in such a way that different layers of the fascial bed of the upper cervical spine are reached each time.

If this technique is applied precisely, we will be able to influence the muscular and ligamentous microstructures of the suboccipital triangle as well as the large longitudinal layers such as the dura and the large anterior longitudinal ligament of the spine at the same time. Because both of these longitudinal layers are connected to the sacrum, I recommend reexamining the sacrum, in particular the second segment of the sacrum, and treating it with the technique described above, if necessary.

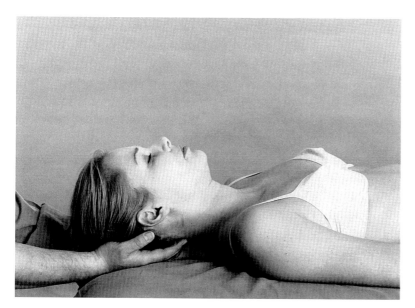

Figure 8.9   Treatment of the transition between the upper chest cavity and lower cervical region.

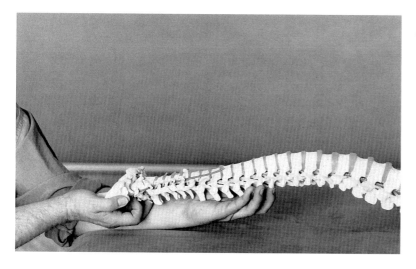

Figure 8.10   Position of the hands, clarified on the skeleton.

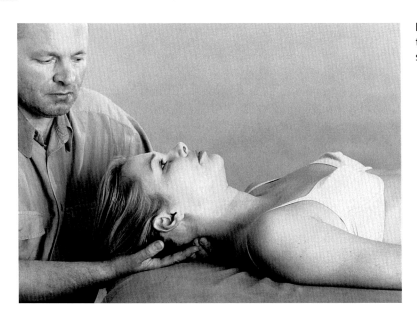

Figure 8.11 Treatment of the transition between the upper cervical spine and the head.

Chapter 9

Treatment after pregnancy and birth

Pregnancy and the birth of a child cause long-term changes to a woman's entire myofascial system. The increase in volume of the pelvic cavity produces a drastic shear effect in the cranial direction and on the organs located below the diaphragm. At the same time, the pressure increases in the inferior direction and in the lateral direction on both sides. Owing to hormonal influences, the tensile force of the ligaments decreases during advanced pregnancy, which is an essential condition for a problem-free birth. However, because the tensile force of the ligaments is still reduced months after birth, lasting changes can develop in the joint system.

Changes occur in the fascial layers of the lower extremities as well. In order to counteract the weight of the child, the tone of the musculature on the posterior side of the legs must increase, usually first in the lower legs. The gastrocnemius and soleus muscles are particularly affected. Because the increase in muscle tone is effective over a period of months, the fascial sheath layers of the affected muscles react with corresponding reinforcement and orientation of their fibers. This process also causes aftereffects that are significant for months after birth.

The change in position by the organs in the pelvic and abdominal cavities during pregnancy is only possible because the peritoneum changes as well; its surface increases by far more than its regular area of $2\,m^2$. This process also has consequences that reach far beyond the pregnancy. Only some of the excess peritoneal layers are able to degenerate on their own after birth.

It is characteristic of the process of change that occurs during pregnancy that precisely localized detailed fixations as well as large-area layers of the parietal system are influenced. In the case of first pregnancies, it is entirely possible that the increased effects of force inside the abdominal and pelvic cavities may release fixations. Pregnancy is, after all, a natural process and this process has a great positive potential for the correction of the inner structure of the myofascial system. It is precisely for this reason that it is necessary to proceed in a very targeted manner with corrective treatment impulses after birth. The woman's organism has completed a far-reaching conversion process and many tissue layers are in a rather hypotonic state. Therefore, the therapist's job is merely to treat a few restrictions of motion as carefully as possible and otherwise influence the overall form of the organism with globally applied techniques in such a way that the natural regeneration process can occur without a problem.

Treatment of shortened myofascial layers in the region of the lower leg

Patient Prone, both legs extended, arms resting to the side of the torso.

Therapist Standing at the feet.

Contact With the middle phalanges of one hand at the transition between the Achilles tendon and the distal end of the gastrocnemius muscle, the second hand supports the lower leg from the anterior direction in the region of the tibialis anterior.

Action The therapist supports one knee on the lower end of the treatment table and the therapist's thigh supports the toes and transverse arch of the foot. The patient's knee is slightly bent. Using the surface of the middle phalanges of one hand, the therapist first applies pressure to the superficial layer of the crural fascia in order to then apply pressure at a very oblique angle almost parallel to the skin to the superficial and middle layers of the gastrocnemius and soleus muscles. The other hand supports the lower leg from the anterior direction with firm contact on the anterior portion of the fasciae. While the contact is maintained in the anterior region without any sliding, the therapist exerts a stretching push in the posterior section, sliding at the contact point very slowly and only a few centimeters. The therapist then asks the patient to push the knee gently into the treatment table and stretch the heel somewhat. It is crucial that the sliding on the posterior side of the thigh be conducted very slowly and the intensity of the contact be maintained during the entire sequence of movements.

This technique should then be applied analogously to the other leg. We have to pay close attention to the differences between sides and modify the angle of application and intensity of pressure correspondingly.

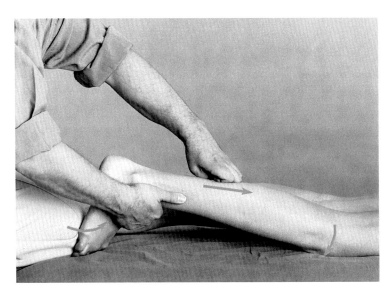

Figure 9.1 Treatment of shortened myofascial layers in the region of the lower leg.

Treatment of the myofascial tension patterns of the thigh

Patient Prone, both legs extended, arms resting to the side of the torso.

Therapist Standing at the level of the knees.

Contact One hand supports the thigh from the anterior direction while the other hand reaches between the biceps femoris and semitendinosus muscle from the posterior direction above the knee.

Action The therapist supports the thigh with one hand in such a way as to produce a flat contact with the anterior layer of the fascia lata parallel to the outside shape. The therapist holds the entire leg so that approximately horizontal hinge axes manifest at the ankle, knee, and hip joint. With the other hand, the therapist reaches parallel to the orientation of the muscle fibers between the muscle bellies of the long head of the biceps femoris and the semitendinosus muscle. The therapist uses his or her body weight to allow the touch to first sink through the superficial layer and then make contact between the fascial sheaths of the two muscle bellies. The therapist selects the direction of pressure in such a way that the tissue is not crushed against the bone located below it. With intensive contact, the therapist gradually moves in the proximal direction toward the ischial tuberosity.

This technique is then applied in an analogous manner for the fascial boundary layers between the adductor magnus and semitendinosus muscles as well as on the other leg. It may be necessary to modify this technique in relation to existing tension conditions.

The technique described for the lower leg and thigh can be applied in a modified form to any longitudinal muscles of the posterior side of the leg. For the efficacy of this technique, it is necessary to create an intensive contact with the fasciae and to ensure that the pressure actually reaches the fascial layer between the muscle bellies. Any tugging, gliding motion on the skin must be avoided. In addition to this technique, which is applied to a large area, the techniques described in the chapter on the lower extremity can be used as well (see section 4.5, Lower extremity).

Treatment of the fascia of the transversus abdominis and the spatial relationship between intraperitoneal and retroperitoneal components

Patient Sitting upright on a stool with the knee joints at a lower level than the hip joints.

Therapist Kneeling in front of the patient.

Contact With the palms completely relaxed on both sides of the abdominal wall just below the navel.

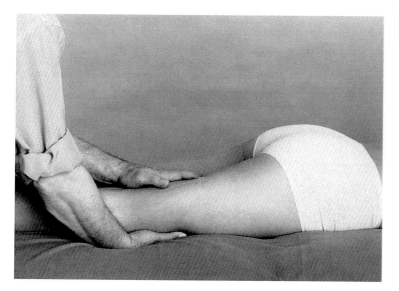

Figure 9.2 Treatment of the myofascial tension patterns of the thigh.

Action   First, the therapist asks the patient to make good contact between both feet and the floor. Then the therapist asks the patient to completely relax the abdominal wall and allow the pelvis to tilt slightly in the anterior direction around the axis of the hips so that the pelvic segment moves toward the therapist's palms. The patient should keep the sternum in a superior–anterior position, but still remain completely relaxed on the anterior side of the body.

The therapist then modifies the contact with both hands as if to carefully support the contents of the pelvis while it tilts forward, and then lifts it minimally in the cranial direction and gradually guides it somewhat farther inward in the direction of the middle central line of the torso. Seen from the outside, it appears as if the therapist were trying to push the organs from both sides toward the front of the spine.

If this technique is correctly applied, a gradual correction of the spatial relationships occurs between the fascial layers of the abdominal wall, the anterior layer of the peritoneum, and the posterior layer of the peritoneum relative to the renal fascia.

The effects of this technique occur gradually. In the weeks after the birth, it acts on the exterior myofascial structure of the pelvic and abdominal cavities and the mobility of the organs. Ultimately, its objective is to move the spread-out parts of the enlarged peritoneum more strongly together and thus allow an improved alignment of the organs of the torso.

This technique consists of active and passive components, which must be taken into account if the technique is to be performed successfully. The tilt of the pelvis in the anterior direction corresponds to the active part; we move our hands only minimally in the dorsal direction. This has an effect on the patient's body as if we were raising the entire contents of the pelvis slightly in the cranial direction. However, this procedure has a passive component as well: in "listening," during the lifting process, we note any resistances that may occur in the tissue. We feel our way layer by layer, first through the muscular fascial structure of the exterior abdominal wall until we reach the transversus

abdominis and its fascia. Only then do we intensify the quality of the touch far enough that the contact encroaches on the peritoneum on both sides. Finally, we allow the touch to act farther in the dorsal direction through the peritoneal cavity until we have the impression that we have arrived at the posterior layer of the peritoneum. In an ideal case, while the patient's pelvic cavity is leaning against our hands, we reach the retroperitoneal cavity just below the kidneys. At this moment, it is worthwhile to change the quality of the touch again in the sense of a very subtle "listening." We may be able to notice a shear effect manifesting on one side in the inferior direction. We follow this effect minimally in the inferior direction and then intensify the impulse gently in the cranial direction.

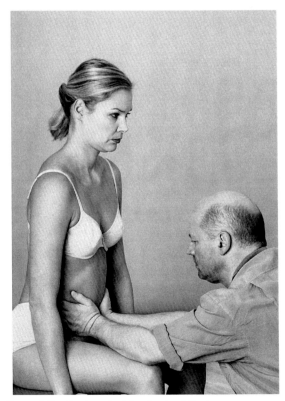

Figure 9.3   Treatment of the fascia of the transversus abdominis and the spatial relationship between intraperitoneal and retroperitoneal components.

Summarizing aspects

Because the movement of the diaphragm is generally limited during pregnancy, lasting changes may also occur to joints in the upper body that are dependent on the movement of the diaphragm. In such cases, before applying the techniques in the lower extremities and the pelvic and abdominal cavities, I recommend ensuring that no articular restrictions are present in the region of the thorax. The costovertebral joints and the sternoclavicular joints require particular attention in these situations (see sections 4.1 and 5.1).

In the gymnastics of regeneration, we must keep in mind that the large changes during pregnancy do not manifest on the actual musculature, but rather on and in the fasciae of the myofascial system. Schematically conducted training of the abdominal muscles may cause the increased area of the peritoneum that is still present to be extended further, or ligaments connected to organs to be overextended. It is advisable to perform exercises for strengthening the muscles only once the ligamentous and membranous layers of the abdominal and pelvic cavities have regained their normal state, which will happen three months after delivery at the earliest. However, there are limitations to strength training of some muscle groups even then, if the coordination of overlapping muscle pulls is not taken into account.

Concluding remarks

For psychologists who have had little education in anatomy, there is sometimes the danger of overlooking the fact that the physical side of a person has its own dynamics. Therefore, overinterpretations of physical expression may occur in psychotherapy. On the other hand, a therapist following a manual approach has the far greater risk of blindly believing in the laws of matter. However, a bent back is not only a pronounced kyphosis of the thoracic spine; it is also an expression of a bent person.

The spatial form of the fascial and membrane network can be read like the story of a person given shape. Recurring motion sequences, the preferred orientation and perception, as well as the prevailing basic emotional pattern, leave their marks on the tissue and can be read there. Thus, a shape develops that is more than a collection of discrete anatomical parts. In the treatment of the fasciae and membranes, the therapist communicates with this shape. Anatomical knowledge is helpful, but it serves more as topographical orientation than as the actual therapeutic technique.

A great virtuoso of the violin once said, "The best technique is the kind that you don't even notice."

I think that what he meant was that efficient technique is applied inconspicuously and is never an end in itself. It is in this spirit that *Fascial and Membrane Technique* addresses the organism as a structure of form. It is applied to the physical structure in order to reach the psychological unity of the person.

Bibliography

Abehsera A. (2000) Craniosacrale Osteopathie: Ein wichtiger Baustein der Osteopathie. *Osteopathische Medizin*, 1.

Abehsera A. (2002) Craniosacrale Osteopathie unter der Lupe—Teil II. *Osteopathische Medizin*, 4.

Barral J-P. (1993) *Manipulations Uro-Genitales*. Éditions de Verlaque: Aix-en-Provence.

Barral J-P. (1996) *Manual Thermal Diagnosis*. Eastland Press: Seattle, WA.

Barral J-P. (2002) *Lehrbuch der viszeralen Osteopathie*. Vol. 2. Urban & Fischer: Jena.

Barral J-P and Croibier A. (1999) *Trauma. An Osteopathic Approach*. Eastland Press: Seattle, WA.

Barral J-P and Croibier A. (2005) *Manipulation peripherer Nerven. Osteopathische Diagnostile und Therapie*. Elsevier: München.

Barral J-P and Mercier P. (1988) *Visceral Manipulation*. Eastland Press: Seattle, WA.

Barral J-P and Mercier P. (2002) *Lehrbuch der viszeralen Osteopathie*. Vol. 1. Urban & Fischer: Jena. A second edition in translation of Barral and Mercier (1988), above.

Barral J-P, Mathieu P and Mercier P. (1993) Die Untersuchung der Wirbelsäule. In *Handbuch für die Osteopathie*. The International Academy of Osteopathy: Gent.

Benninghoff A. (1994) *Anatomie*. Vol. 1, 15th edn. Urban & Schwarzenberg, Munich.

Benninghoff A. (1934) Über die Anordnung und die Bedeutung der Bindgewebssysteme im Gefüge der Muskulatur. *Verhandlungen der Anatomischen Gesellschaft*, 42.

van den Berg F. (ed.) (1999) *Angewandte Physiologie*. Vol. 1: Das Bindegewebe des Bewegungsapparates verstehen und beeinflussen. Thieme: Stuttgart.

Bienfait M. (1982) *Les Fascias*. Societé d'édition Medicale "Le Pousse": Bordeaux.

Boebel R. (1957) Über die Beziehungen des M. iliopsoas mittels seiner Faszie zu den Gefäßen der Fossa iliopectinea. *Zeitschrift für Anatomische Entwicklungsgeschichte*, 120.

Breul R. (2002) Die Blätter der Fascia renalis. *Osteopathische Medizin*, 2.

Croibier A. (2005) *Diagnostic Ostéopathic Général*. Elsevier: Paris.

Friedlin M. (2003) Annäherungen an den Faszienbegriff—Eine semantische Untersuchung. *Osteopathische Medizin*, 1.

Flury H and Harder W. (1988) The tilt of the pelvis. *Notes on Structural Integration*, Zurich, 1.

Godard H. (2003) Verbesserung der sensorischen Dynamik. In Schwind P (ed.) *Alles im Lot. Eine Einführung in die Rolfingmethode*. Droemer-Knaur: Munich.

Heine H. (1997) *Lehrbuch der biologischen Medizin. Grundregulation und extrazellulare Matrix. Grundlagen und Systematik*. 2nd edn. Thieme: Stuttgart.

Horwitz G. (1981) Pneumatic and tensile structures. The work of Frei Otto. *Bulletin of Structural Integration*, 7 (2).

Ingber D. (1998) Architekturen des Lebens. *Spektrum der Wissenschaft*, 3.

Jones LH. (1981) *Strain and Counterstrain*. American Academy of Osteopathy: Newark, NJ.

Kleinau A. (n.d.) Lang- und mittelfristige Ergebnisse nach Operationen wegen eines Karpaltunnelsyndroms. Unpublished manuscript and research report.

Köpf-Maier PS. (2000) *Wolf Heideggers Atlas der Anatomie des Menschen*, 5th edn. 2 vols. Karger: Basel.

von Lanz T and Wachsmuth W. (1972) *Praktische Anatomie. Ein Lehr- und Hilfsbuch der anatomischen Grundlagen ärztlichen Handelns*. 1 vol. Part 4. Springer: Heidelberg.

Lanz U. (1967) Anatomical variations of the median nerve in the carpal tunnel. *Journal of Hand Surgery*, 147.

Liem T. (1998) *Kraniosakrale Osteopathie. Ein praktisches Lehrbuch*. Thieme: Stuttgart.

Liem T. (2000) *Praxis der kraniosakralen Osteopathie*. Thieme: Stuttgart.

Megele E. (1991) Diagnostische Tests beim Karpaltunnelsyndrom. *Der Nervenarzt*, 62.

Meert GF. (2003) *Das Becken aus osteopathischer Sicht. Funktionelle Zusammenhänge nach dem Tensegrity-Modell*. Urban & Fischer: Munich.

Maitland J. (2001) *Spinal Manipulation Made Simple. A Manual of Soft Tissue Techniques*. North Atlantic Books: Berkeley, CA.

Myers T. (2001) *Anatomy Trains. Myofascial Meridians for Manual and Movement Therapists*. Churchill Livingston: Edinburgh.

Morton DJ. (1952) *Human Locomotion and Bodyform. A Study of Gravity and Man*. The Williams & Williams Company: Baltimore, MD.

Müller H. (1990) Morphologische Grundlagen der Kiefergelenksfunktion und deren Störungen und Konsequenzen für Diagnostik und Therapie. Professorial dissertation, Ludwig-Maximillians-Universität, Munich.

Mumenthaler M. (1962) Über Lähmungen peripherer Nerven im Extremitätenbereich. *Deutsche Medizinische Wochenschrift*, 38.

Mumenthaler M. (1964) Die Therapie des Carpaltunnelsyndroms. *Deutsche Medizinische Wochenschrift*, 51.

Mumenthaler M and Schlack H. (eds.) (1982) *Läsionen peripherer Nerven*. 4th edn. Thieme: Stuttgart.

Oschman JL. (2000) *Energy Medicine. The Scientific Basis*. Churchill Livingstone: London.

Pernkopf E. (1987) *Atlas der topographischen und angewandten Anatomie des Menschen*, 2nd edn. Ed. H Fermer. Urban u. Schwarzenberg: Munich.

Paoletti S. (2001) *Faszien. Anatomie—Strukturen—Techniken— Spezielle Osteopathie*. Urban & Fischer: Munich.

Prat D. (1993) Le cadre osteo-musculaire de la sphere uro-genitale. In Prat D et al. *Nouvelles Techniques urogenitales*. Éditions de Verlaque: Aix-en-Provence.

Prat D. (1999) Manual diagnostics. Lecture at the interdisciplinary symposium by the Munich Group, Villa Degiani, Friuli.

Rauber A and Kopsch F. (1987) *Anatomie des Menschen. Lehrbuch und Atlas*. Ed. H Leonhardt, B Tillmann, G Töndury and K Zilles. Thieme: Stuttgart.

Rolf IP. (1993) *Rolfing im Überblick*. Junfermann: Paderborn.

Rolf IP. (1997) *Rolfing—Strukturelle Integration. Wandel und Gleichgewicht der Körperstruktur*. Ed. and rev. P Schwind. 2nd edn. Irisiana: Munich.

Schleip R. (2003) Faszien und Nervensystem. *Osteopathische Medizin*, vol. 1.

Schleip R, Klinger W and Lehmann-Horn F. (2005) Active fascial contractility: Fascia is able to actively contract and relax in a smooth muscle like manner and thereby influence biomechanical behavior. *Acta Physiologica*, 186 (Suppl. 1).

Schulz L and Feitis R. (1996) *The Endless Web. Fascial Anatomy and Physical Reality*. North Atlantic Books: Berkeley, CA.

Schwind P. (2003) *Alles im Lot. Eine Einführung in die Rolfingmethode*. Droemer-Knaur: Munich.

Schwind P. (2001) Die manuelle Behandlung des Karpaltunnelsyndroms—Faszien- und Membrantechnik. *Osteopathische Medizin*, 3.

Schwind P. (2002) Faszientechnik für Behandlung des Kiefergelenks. *Osteopathische Medizin*, 1.

Sobotta J. (2001) *Atlas der Anatomie des Menschen*, 21st edn. 2 vols. Ed. R Putz and R Pabst. Urban & Fischer: Munich.

Staubesand J and Li Y. (1996) Zum Feinbau der Fascia cruris unter Berücksichtigung epi- und intrafaszialer Nerven. *Manuelle Medizin*, Springer: Berlin, 34 (5).

Sutherland WG. (1990) *Teachings in the Science of Osteopathy*. Ed. A Wales. Rudra Press: Portland, OR.

Tittel K. (1978) *Beschreibende und funktionelle Anatomie des Menschen*. 8th edn. Gustav Fischer: Stuttgart.

Upledger JE and Vredevoogd JD. (1983) *Craniosacral Therapy*. Eastland Press: Seattle, WA.

Varela FJ and Frank S. (1987) The organ of form: toward a theory of biological shape. *Journal of Social and Biological Structures*, 10.

Waldeyer A and Mayet A. (1993) *Anatomie des Menschen*, 16th edn. 2 vols. De Gruyter: Berlin.

Wilhelm K. (1987) Kompressionssyndrome des Nervus ulnaris und Nervus medianus im Handbereich, *Orthopäde*, 16.

Zumhasch R and Hinz C. (1999) *Das Karpaltunnelsyndrom. Anatomie, Ätiologie, Diagnostik und präoperative und postoperative Behandlungsmöglichkeiten*. Part I: *Ergotherapie & Rehabilitation*, 5.

Index

Note: page numbers in *italics* refer to figures and tables.

Printed in the United States
By Bookmasters